Substance Abuse and Mental Health Practice

Substance Abuse and Mental Health Practice

A Casebook on Co-Occurring Disorders

Cognella Casebook Series for the Human Services

Jerry L. Johnson and George Grant, Jr.

Grand Valley State University

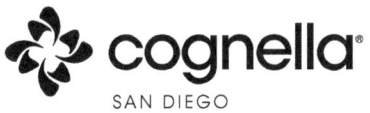

SAN DIEGO

Bassim Hamadeh, CEO and Publisher
Amy Smith, Senior Project Editor
Alia Bales, Production Editor
Jess Estrella, Senior Graphic Designer
Stephanie Kohl, Licensing Coordinator
Natalie Piccotti, Director of Marketing
Kassie Graves, Vice President of Editorial
Jamie Giganti, Director of Academic Publishing

Copyright © 2021 by Cognella, Inc. All rights reserved. No part of this publication may be reprinted, reproduced, transmitted, or utilized in any form or by any electronic, mechanical, or other means, now known or hereafter invented, including photocopying, microfilming, and recording, or in any information retrieval system without the written permission of Cognella, Inc. For inquiries regarding permissions, translations, foreign rights, audio rights, and any other forms of reproduction, please contact the Cognella Licensing Department at rights@cognella.com.

Trademark Notice: Product or corporate names may be trademarks or registered trademarks and are used only for identification and explanation without intent to infringe.

Cover image Copyright © 2016 Depositphotos/Syda_Productions.

Printed in the United States of America.

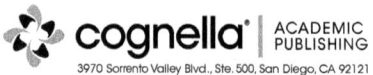

To my wonderful parents, Lee and Joanne Johnson, who continue to encourage and support me in my endeavors. You are the best parents a man could have.

Jerry L. Johnson

To my wife, Beverly, who inspires and supports me in all my endeavors. In loving memory of my father and mother, George and Dorothy Grant.

George Grant, Jr.

BRIEF CONTENTS

Preface xv

1 A Multiple Systems Approach to Practice with Co-Occurring Disorders 1

2 Jeremiah Cartwright 33

3 Juan or John 63

4 Sara 91

5 Appearances Can Be Deceiving 111

6 Meet James Snyder 135

7 Co-Occurring Disorders Treatment 161

About the Editors 185

About the Authors 187

DETAILED CONTENTS

Preface xv

1   A Multiple Systems Approach to Practice with Co-Occurring Disorders   1
   Jerry L. Johnson
   Advanced Multiple Systems (AMS) Practice   2
      Sociological Roots   2
   AMS Overview   4
      Multiple Systems Perspective   4
   Dimensions of AMS Assessment   7
      A. Dimension 1: Client Description, Presenting Problem, and Referral   7
      B. Dimension 2: Treatment/Therapy History   7
      C. Dimension 3: Substance Use History   7
      D. Dimension 4: Mental Health History   8
      E. Dimension 5: Family History   8
      F. Dimension 6: Social Support and Engagement   9
      G. Dimension 7: Culture   9
      H. Dimension 8: Biopsychosocial Connection   9
   Guiding Practice Principles   10
   Guiding Practice Principles Explained   11
      First Principle (Umbrella Principle): Healthy Outcomes (and Lives) are Directly Related to People's Connections to Helpful, Supportive Systems, Across a Lifetime   11
      Client Engagement   14
      Fostering, Building, or Rediscovering Hopes and Dreams   16
      Principle A: Clients Are People, Too   19
      Principle B: Check Your Practice/Professional Privilege at the Door   20
      Structural and Historical Systems of Privilege and Oppression: Who Holds the Power?   20
      Principle C: Culturally Respectful and Responsive Client Engagement   22
      Principle D: Motivation Matters   25

1. *Precontemplation* 26
　　　2. *Contemplation Stage* 28
　　　3. *Preparation Stage* 28
　　　4. *Action Stage* 29
　　　5. *Maintenance Stage* 29
　　　6. *Relapse Stage* 29
　　　Last Principle: When All Else Fails, Never Do Anything That Violates the First Principle! 30
　　Summary 30
　　Core Beliefs 30
　　References 31

2　Jeremiah Cartwright 33
　　Jerry L. Johnson
　　Jeremiah's Situation at Referral 33
　　Working with Mandated Clients 34
　　Our First Meeting 36
　　　The Shooting and Its Immediate Aftermath 39
　　　Treatment History 40
　　Session Two: Alcohol and Drugs 44
　　　Jeremiah's Extended Family 45
　　　Fiona's Extended Family 47
　　　Jeremiah and Fiona 48
　　　Drinking and Legal History 50
　　Session Three: Turning Point 53
　　　Dealing with Jeremiah's Intoxication 54
　　　Jeremiah's Major Conflict 57
　　Case Summary 58
　　Assessment, Diagnoses, and Treatment Planning 59
　　Intervention Planning and Implementation 60
　　Termination, Aftercare, and Follow-Up 61
　　References 61

3　Juan or John 63
　　Salvador Lopez-Arias
　　Introduction 63
　　Meeting Juan (Or John) 64
　　　What's in a Name? John or Juan? 66
　　Approaching John in Therapy 68
　　　Our Work Begins: John and Lisa's Marriage 71
　　　Domestic Violence 72

    Religion   76
    John's Family of Origin   77
  John Returns   80
  Session Three and Beyond   84
    Mental Health Screening and Observations   84
  Case Summary   87
  Assessment, Diagnoses, and Treatment Planning   88
  References   88

4 Sara   91
  Carolyn Sutherby
  Introduction   91
  Sara: Case Background   91
  Meeting Sara   92
  Context of Her Referral for an Assessment   94
  Sara's Family History   96
  Mental Health History   97
  Family Mental Health History   99
  Medical and Medication History   99
  Substance Use History   102
  Case Comments   107
  References   110

5 Appearances Can Be Deceiving   111
  Salvador Lopez-Arias and Jerry L. Johnson
  Introduction   111
  Substance Abuse Assessment   113
    A. Brief Description of Client   113
    B. Chief Complaint and Symptoms by Client and Others Present   114
    C. Context of the Referral, Precipitating Events, Facts, and Dates   114
    Treatment History   115
    Substance Use History   117
    Medical History   122
    Basic Needs   123
    Mental Health, Psychological and Emotional Functioning   123
    Emotional Functioning   124
    Mental Health Status, Psychological and Emotional Function Narrative   125
    Family History   128
    Cultural/Spiritual Context (Racial Identity, Oppression/

        Discrimination)   *130*
        Social-Relational and Social Support   *131*
    Narrative Assessment   133
        Treatment Plan   *133*
        Treatment Recommendation   *133*
        Goals   *133*
        High-Risk Aftercare and Intervention Plan   *134*
    Reference   134

6   Meet James Snyder   135
    Jerry L. Johnson
    Introduction   135
    Substance Use and Mental Health Assessment   137
        A. Brief Description of Client   *137*
        B. Chief Complaint and Symptoms by Client and Others   *137*
        C. Context of the Referral, Precipitating Events, Facts, and Dates   *138*
        Substance Use and/or Mental Health Treatment History   *139*
        Substance Use History   *141*
        Medical History   *144*
        Basic Needs   *145*
        Mental Health Status   *146*
        Mental Status Impressions (Potential Mood, Anxiety, Thought, or Personality Disorders)   *149*
        Family History and Structure   *150*
        Social Support and Engagement   *152*
        Legal History   *153*
        Cultural Background and Engagement   *154*
        Treatment Plan   *157*
        Treatment Recommendation   *157*
        Goals   *157*
        High-Risk Aftercare and Intervention Plan   *158*
    Reference   159

7   Co-Occurring Disorders Treatment   161
    Jerry L. Johnson and Glen Brookhouse
    Introduction   161
    Overview   161
    Treating Co-Occurring Disorders in Single-Focus Substance Abuse Programs   163
    Current Best Practices   164

Integrated Care　164
　　　The Four Quadrants of Care　167
　　　Treatment Models and Methods: Current Findings　169
　　　Level and Intensity of Care　173
　Best-Practice Treatment Recommendations　173
　Core Beliefs　178
　References　179

About the Editors　185

About the Authors　187

PREFACE

WELCOME TO OUR new Casebook Series for the Human Services. This series of books is designed to improve professional practice education across the human services. As the editors, we are thrilled by our partnership with Cognella to make these books available to educators and students across the human services spectrum.

This text, *Substance Abuse and Mental Health Practice: A Casebook on Co-Occurring Disorders*, will enhance the clinical preparation of students and practitioners across the helping professions, who are either presently working with this population or interested in doing so in the future.

As graduate and undergraduate social work educators, we (Johnson and Grant) understand the struggle to find quality clinical practice materials that translate well into a classroom setting. In the past, we used case materials from our practice careers. Then, in the early 2000s we edited and published the Allyn & Bacon Casebook Series between 2005 and 2007. The original Casebook Series covered eight different practice areas (substance abuse, mental health, domestic violence, sexual abuse, adoption, foster care, community practice, and medical social work).

While we were happy with the first series, we wanted to improve its quality and usefulness in the classroom while updating the topics to more closely match current trends. Over the years, we sought and received extensive feedback from readers and faculty adopters about the strengths and weaknesses of the previous series. Most importantly, we asked specific questions about each case's ease of use in the classroom.

In preparing the new series, we relied heavily on feedback, resulting in the book you are reading, and forthcoming Casebooks in the series. We believe the new Casebook Series for the Human Services, as evidenced by this text, published by our friends at Cognella, achieved our goal of enhanced learning opportunities and ease of classroom use.

Our goal is always to give student readers the chance to study, assess, and analyze how experienced practitioners think about practice, struggle to resolve practice dilemmas, and make clinical decisions to meet the needs of their clients. We believe the structure of our cases, written in narrative voice and story format, allows readers access to the minds of experienced practitioners in a way that will improve engagement, assessment, diagnostic, and treatment planning skills, but more importantly, enhance the way students think about their clients and practice.

Overall, we intend for the Casebook Series for the Human Services to provide a learning experience that:

1. Provides readers an overview of our previously published Advanced Multiple Systems (AMS) approach to practice (Johnson & Grant, 2005). This practice perspective describes an approach to practice as both a simple guide to working the cases in the Casebooks and for later in their practice careers.

    More importantly, we define AMS through a series of Guiding Practice Principles, developed by the editors over the course of long careers, study, and experience. Our Guiding Practice Principles offer a way for practitioners to think about and act in practice settings to help guide successful engagement leading to a positive helping experience for clients and professionals.
2. Offers personal and intimate glimpses into the thinking and actions of experienced practitioners as they work with diverse clients across different practice settings. In working through each case, students have the chance to demonstrate their understanding of the clinical and social issues presented while learning to use high-level "assessment thinking" through the various questions and exercises included to help make sense of each case.
3. Provides multiple opportunities to develop comprehensive clinical assessments, diagnoses, treatment plans, and emergency plans for a variety of presenting problems from a diverse client group. These exercises also provide excellent opportunities for large and small group discussions to enhance the learning experience. The cases are also well-suited for use in online and remote courses.
4. Offers students and readers an up-to-date critical review of Best Practice Methods for the practice area in each book. The final chapter of each book will guide readers through the professional literature and evidence-based research to provide an extensive review of current practice trends in the field of study.

As former practitioners, we chose the cases carefully. Each case making the "cut" focuses on the process (thinking, planning, and decision-making) of practice and not necessarily on techniques or outcomes. We chose cases based on one simple criterion: did it provide the best possible opportunity for excellence in practice education? We asked authors to "teach practice" by considering cases that were interesting and difficult, regardless of outcome, and to let readers into their internal thought processes as their case progressed.

In addition, each case focuses on client engagement and cultural responsiveness as important aspects of the practice process. As we like to remind our social work students, there are two words in the title of the profession: *social* and *work*. For the "work" to occur, students must learn to master the "social"—primarily, client engagement and relationship building in a culturally inviting and responsive manner.

As you will learn in Chapter 1, practice is relationship based and, from our perspective, relies more on the processes involved in relationship building and client engagement than technical intervention skills. Successful practice is often rooted more in the ability of practitioners to develop open and trusting relationships with client(s) than on their ability to employ specific methods of intervention.

Yet, this critically important element of practice is often ignored or only mentioned in passing as a given. Our experience with students, employees, and practitioner/trainees over nearly four decades suggests it is wrong to assume students and/or practitioners have competent engagement or relationship-building skills. Developing a professional relationship based in trust and openness, where clients feel safe to dialogue about the most intimate and sometimes embarrassing events in their lives, is the primary responsibility of the practitioner. Hence, each case presentation tries to provide a sense of this difficult and often elusive process, along with ways each author managed the emerging client relationship.

TARGET AUDIENCE

We believe this series is applicable and useful for education and training programs from community college, to advanced undergraduate, and graduate programs in the helping professions. We also know of many social agencies that provide our previous texts to new employees for review and practice. Hence, the Casebooks are appropriate in social work, counseling psychology, counseling, mental health, psychology, and specialty disciplines such as marriage and family therapy, substance abuse, and mental health degree or certificate programs. Any educational or training program designed to prepare students to work with clients in a helping capacity may find the Casebooks useful as a learning tool.

STRUCTURE OF CASES

There are two different case formats in this book. In Chapters 2, 3, and 4, each case is presented as an in-depth narrative written as a story. The authors provide an inside look into actual therapy sessions as they build rapport, develop client engagement, and make decisions about how best to gather personal information leading to an accurate assessment, diagnoses, and treatment plan. These stories often include client-practitioner dialogue to help readers gaze inside a confidential therapy session and periodically explore practice literature to explain certain dilemmas as they arise in the case.

The narrative case studies are designed to maximize critical thinking, the use of professional literature, evidenced-based practice knowledge, and classroom discussion in the learning process. At various points throughout each case, the editors include a series of thought-provoking and/or action-based questions to guide and enhance the learning process. We want readers to collect evidence on different sides of an issue, evaluate that evidence, and develop a professional position they can defend in writing and/or discussion with other students in the classroom or seminar setting.

Chapters 5 and 6 in this text use a different case study format, albeit the cases are still presented in depth. In these cases, author(s) completed intake and assessment interviews and compiled the client information on a standard comprehensive assessment form, minus clinical conclusions, meaning, or summaries. Those sections of the assessment form are left blank. Readers are asked to read and understand the client information and complete each section of the assessment that requires "assessment thinking": that is, develop appropriate clinical conclusions, meaning, and summaries as required.

At the end of each case, readers can develop a comprehensive narrative assessment based on the client's information, accurate clinical diagnoses, appropriate treatment plan, and an emergency/safety plan. Moreover, readers are asked to determine the client's stage of change (see Chapter 1) for each clinical diagnosis. Cases in this format make for excellent in-class exercises that teach both clinical decision making and professional assessment writing.

We hope that you find the cases and our formats as instructive and helpful in your courses, as we have in ours. We have field tested these two formats in our courses, finding that students respond well to the length, depth, and rigor of the case presentations.

ORGANIZATION OF THIS TEXT

We organized this book on Practice with Co-Occurring Disorders to maximize its utility in any course. Chapter 1 provides an overview of our Advanced Multiple Systems (AMS) practice approach, focusing on a series of Guiding Practice Principles gleaned from the editors' nearly 80 years of combined professional experience. The AMS is one potential organizing tool for students to use while reading and evaluating the cases.

The Guiding Practice Principles provide important ways of thinking and approaching clients in all practice settings to help the engagement, assessment, and treatment process. These principles are not connected to theory, method, or practice setting/role. Similar to a professional code of ethics, the Guiding Practice Principles offer critical elements for effective clinical and relationship decisions.

In Chapter 2, Jerry L. Johnson tells the narrative story of the first three therapy sessions with **Jeremiah Cartwright**, an Iraq War veteran. Over the course of this chapter, Jeremiah's war-related struggles and his efforts to cope while maintaining his role as husband and father become apparent as the story progresses. This chapter focuses in detail about the struggles of engaging a mandated client experiencing both substance use and mental health disorders.

In Chapter 3, Salvador Lopez-Arias presents **John or Juan: A Case of Lost Racial Identity**. In this clinical story-based case study, Lopez-Arias demonstrates the negative effects of John/Juan's personal life, health, and racial identity living as a stigmatized racial minority while struggling to "pass" as a member of the majority in the United States.

In Chapter 4, entitled **Sara: Trauma, Mental Health, Substance Abuse, and Parental Rights**, Dr. Carolyn Sutherby provides an in-depth look into the life and world of Sara, as she navigates her life of substance use and trauma, in the context of an active Child Protective Services investigation, fighting to retain custody of her children.

In Chapter 5, Jerry L. Johnson and Salvador Lopez-Arias present the case **Appearances Can Be Deceiving: The Case of Mark Johnson**. In this case, the authors present a look inside the life of Mark Johnson, a Harvard-educated, successful businessman struggling to survive a lifetime of hidden problems. The authors provide Mark's life information on a standard client assessment form, leaving it to readers to make clinical sense of his complex life.

In Chapter 6, **Meet James Snyder: The Wonder Boy with Secrets**, the author describes a case of a local "hero" whose grip on his local Wonder Boy is tenuous. As in the previous chapter, the author provides readers with James's life information on a standard client assessment form, leaving it to readers to make clinical sense of his information and complex life.

In the final chapter, Jerry L. Johnson and Glen Brookhouse provide a comprehensive review of Best Practice Methods in the field of co-occurring disorders. The authors present the current literature and research/evaluation results to determine best practices in the field of co-occurring disorders. The chapter ends with an 11-point list of Best Practice Recommendations.

ACKNOWLEDGMENTS

We would like to thank the contributors to this text for their hard work, experience, and willingness to share their work with our audience. We would also like to thank Amy Smith, Laura Pasquale, and all the professionals at Cognella for being great to work with, for their faith in the Casebook Series for the Human Services, and in our ability to manage multiple manuscripts at once. Additionally, we want to thank our students over the years for serving as "guinea pigs" as we refined our case formats for publication. Their willingness to provide honest feedback contributes mightily to this series.

Jerry L. Johnson: I want to thank my wife, Cheryl, for her support and willingness to give me the time and encouragement to write and edit. I also thank my equine herd—Joey, Hope, Zelda, Ruby, Pip, Rome, Bray, Tommy, Mister Mule, Hershey, Maddy, and Oprah—for helping provide peace in my life.

George Grant, Jr.: I dedicate this book and all my work to my wife, Beverly F. Grant. Thank you for your love, support, and encouragement.

REFERENCE

Johnson, J. L., & Grant Jr., G. (2005). *Casebook: Substance abuse.* Allyn & Bacon.

CHAPTER 1

A Multiple Systems Approach to Practice with Co-Occurring Disorders

Jerry L. Johnson

IN THIS TEXT, we help readers build practice knowledge, values, and skills to work with clients presenting with both substance use and mental health disorders, called co-occurring disorders. We define co-occurring disorders as clients presenting with at least one substance use disorder and at least one mental health disorder. While the simultaneous disorders certainly influence and exacerbate each other, to be considered co-occurring disorders, each must exist independent of the other(s). That is, the substance use and mental health disorders cannot be caused by or a side effect of the other (Johnson, 2004), and if one disorder were magically removed, the other would remain as an existing, diagnosable disorder. For example, it is possible for a client to have an alcohol use disorder and an anxiety disorder co-occurring but not if the anxiety symptoms are solely the result of withdrawals from a long-term alcohol use disorder.

The art and science of accurately assessing, diagnosing, and treatment planning with co-occurring disorders clients is difficult at best, given the intertwined nature and common symptomology of both, and the short turnaround time many organizations and funding sources (i.e., private health insurance, etc.) require for reimbursement. Since accurate assessment and diagnosis are crucial if treatment is to be successfully matched to client need (Johnson, 2004), these skills are important to know, understand, and master.

In this text, we provide a rare opportunity to study the processes and strategies involved in meeting, engaging, assessing, and treating unique clients, all with co-occurring disorders, taken from the caseloads of experienced practitioners. We include five cases, each written with deep and rich case detail designed to plunge readers into the thinking, planning, and approaches of the practitioners/authors. We challenge you to study their thinking and methods, to understand their clinical decision making, and then think critically using your own background and experience to discover and propose alternative ways of working with the same clients. In other words, what would you do if you were the primary practitioner responsible for these cases? How would you approach the cases similarly or differently, and what are your reasons for these differences?

Before diving into the cases, this chapter introduces the Advanced Multiple Systems (AMS) practice perspective, along with the Guiding Practice Principles underlying the AMS. We include AMS and its principles for three reasons. First, AMS can be a guide to help assess and analyze the cases in this text. Each case chapter will ask you to complete a multiple systems assessment, diagnoses, treatment, and intervention plan. AMS provides a theoretical and practical approach for these exercises. Second, we hope you find that AMS makes conceptualizing cases clearer in your practice environment. Third, AMS and the practice principles offer an experience-based way of thinking and acting about and with clients across the practice spectrum. The Guiding Practice Principles offer young and experienced practitioners alike a time-tested way to think about and approach clients in clinical and other practice settings, and they provide the foundation on which successful practice rests.

We do not believe AMS is the only way—or necessarily even the best way—for all practitioners to think about clients. We simply know, through experience, that AMS and the Guiding Practice Principles are an effective way to think about practice with clients from diverse backgrounds and with different needs. While there are many approaches to practice, AMS offers an effective way to place clinical decisions in the context of client lives and experiences, giving engagement and treatment a chance to be productive.

ADVANCED MULTIPLE SYSTEMS (AMS) PRACTICE

Sociological Roots

> Whether the point of interest is a high power state or a minor literary mood, a family, a prison, and a creed—these are the kinds of questions the best social analysts have asked. They are the intellectual pivots of classic studies of (person) in society—and they are the questions inevitably raised by any mind possessing the sociological imagination. For that imagination is the capacity to shift from one perspective to another—from the political to the psychological; from an examination of a single-family to comparative assessment of the national budgets of the world; from the theological school to the military establishment; from considerations of an oil industry to studies of contemporary poetry. It is the capacity to range from the most impersonal and remote transformations to the most intimate

features of the human self—and see the relations between the two. Back of its use is always the urge to know the social and historical meaning of the individual in the society and in the period in which he (or she) has his quality and his (or her) being. (Mills, 1959, p. 7; parentheses added)

Above, sociologist C. Wright Mills provided an important description of the sociological imagination. As it turns out, Mills' sociological imagination is also an apt description of AMS. Mills believed that linking people's "private troubles" to "public issues" (p. 2) was the most effective way to understand people and their problems, by placing them in social and historical context. It forces investigators to contextualize individuals and families in the framework of the larger social, political, economic, and historical environments in which they live. Ironically, this is also the goal of clinical practice (Germain & Gitterman, 1996; Longres, 2000). Going further, Mills (1959) states:

> We have come to know that every individual lives, from one generation to the next, in some society; that he (or she) lives out a biography, and that he (or she) lives it out within some historical sequence. By the fact of his (or her) living he (or she) contributes, however minutely, to the shaping of this society and to the course of its history, even as he (or she) is made by society and by its historical push and shove. (p. 6)

Mills (1959) proposed this approach to help understand links between people, their lives, and the larger environment. Yet, while laying the theoretical groundwork for social research, Mills also provided the theoretical foundation for an effective approach to clinical practice. This suggests three relevant points directly related to clinical practice.

1. It is crucial to recognize the relationships between people's personal issues and strengths (private troubles) and the issues (political, economic, social, historical, and legal) and strengths of the multiple systems environment (public issues) in which people live. This includes recognizing and integrating issues and strengths at the micro (individual, family, extended kin, etc.), mezzo (local community), and macro (state, region, national, and international policy, laws, political, economic, and social) levels during client engagement, assessment, treatment and aftercare.
2. Understanding these relationships can lead people toward change. We speak here about second-order change, or a significant change that makes a long-term difference in people's lives; the kind of change that alters the fundamental rules of an existing system, helping people see themselves differently in relationship to their world. Second-order change is often

forced from the outside of the system (or person). This level of change becomes possible when people make links across their world in a way that makes sense to them (Freire, 1993). In other words, clients become "empowered" to change when they understand their life in the context of their world, how often their lives have been limited or defined by that wor and realizing they have previously unknown or unimagined choices in how they live, think, feel, believe, and act.

3. Any assessment, clinical diagnoses, or treatment plan excluding multiple systems links does not provide a holistic picture of people's lives, their troubles, and/or strengths. The opportunity for change lessens when client history is overlooked. A practitioner cannot learn too much about their clients, their lives, and their attitudes, beliefs, and values stemming from their local environment, the influence of important relationships, and their sense of hope for a better future.

AMS OVERVIEW

First, we define the foundational concept, the multiple systems perspective. Understanding these ideas provides the foundation for a common language and idea of the concepts used throughout the remainder of this chapter.

Multiple Systems Perspective

Generally, a systems approach emphasizes the connectedness between people and their problems to the complex interrelationships existing in their world (Timberlake, Farber, & Sabatino, 2002). To explain these connections, systems theory emphasizes three important concepts: wholeness, relationships, and homeostasis.

Wholeness refers to the way various parts or subsystems interact to form a whole. This idea asserts that systems cannot be understood or explained unless the connectedness of the subsystems to the whole are understood; the nature of the relationships within the system and the roles people play within that system. In other words, the whole is greater than the sum of its parts. Moreover, systems theory also posits that change in one subsystem will affect change in the whole system.

Relationship refers to the patterns of interaction and overall structures existing within and between subsystems. The nature of these relationships is more important than the system itself. That is, when trying to understand or explain a system (individual, family, or organization, etc.) how subsystems connect through relationships, the characteristics of the relationships between subsystems, and how the subsystems interact provide clues to understanding the whole and the problems needing treatment.

Hence, the application of systems theory is primarily based on understanding relationships. In systems (families, individuals, etc.), problems occur between people (relationships), not "in" them. Even individual diagnoses are looked at by how they affect self and others, along with how the symptoms and/or behavior is encouraged or maintained by relationships within the system. Hence, from this perspective people's internal problems relate to the nature of the relationships in the systems where they live and interact.

Homeostasis refers to the idea that systems strive to maintain and preserve the existing system, its rules and relationships; the status quo. For example, family members assume roles that serve to protect and maintain family stability, often at the expense of "needed" change, or their own individual health and well-being.

The natural tendency toward homeostasis in systems represents what we call the "dilemma of change," where a dilemma is a series of choices, none of which are obviously good (Johnson, 2004). This is best described as the apparent conflict occurring when clients approach moments of significant change. People struggle with the dilemma of change: should they change, risking the unknown, or try remaining the same, even if the status quo is unhealthy or unproductive?

When individuals within systems change, its forces others within the system to change as well, even if only in relation to the individual trying to change. So, if a mother with a long-term substance use disorder suddenly finds sobriety, her newly found life will require everyone else in the family to change in relation to her, even if they do not want to change. This often starts a series of relationship reactions, sometimes leading to the reinstatement of homeostasis that could come in the form of the mother relapsing to ensure family status quo.

What do we mean, then, by the term **multiple systems**? People (clients) are part of and interact with multiple systems simultaneously. These systems interact on many levels, ranging from the micro level (individual and families), the mezzo level (local community, institutions, organizations, the practitioner and their agency, etc.), to the macro level (culture, laws and policy, politics, oppression and discrimination, international events, etc.). How these various systems come together and interact comprise the "whole" that is the client. The nature of these interactions and relationships often helps explain the nature of a client's problems.

In practice, the client (individual, couple, family, etc.) is not the "system," but one of many interacting subsystems in a maze of other subsystems constantly interacting to create the system—the client plus elements from multiple subsystems at each level. It would be a mistake to view the client as the whole system, or that individual problems are not affected by other aspects of the system (family and beyond).

This level of understanding—the system as the whole produced through multiple system interactions—is the main unit of investigation for practice. As stated above, it is narrow to consider the client as a functioning independent system with peripheral involvement with others existing outside of their intimate world.

These issues and relationships work together to help shape and mold the client who in turn, shapes and molds their relationship to the other subsystems.

For example, an African American teenage student may have every intention of being a top academic performer in his mostly white high school. During class one day, the teacher asks something of the student, leading him to question the teacher on her reasons for asking. In this young man's family and culture, it is not unusual to talk loudly, more loudly than what is often considered "normal" in a white environment.

The student's tone and volume encourage his white teacher to believe the student is being challenging or even threatening, depending on her subjective experience with students of color. The student is immediately sent to the principal's office for "acting out" and being "threatening," although he simply asked for clarification in the ways of his family and culture, but not his teacher's. This student then risks becoming labeled as "oppositional" among the other teachers, who his teacher talks to every day. He also risks being referred for therapy or counseling to treat his "oppositional defiant disorder." In this case, multiple systems interacted against what our fictional student believed and was taught about his right to question and seek clarification about teacher requests. Interacting systems collided to create a problem where none existed.

AMS provides an organized framework for gathering, conceptualizing, and analyzing multiple system client data to help practitioners proceed with the helping process. Beginning with culturally responsive client engagement, a comprehensive multi-systems assessment points toward a holistically based treatment plan that requires practitioners to select and utilize appropriate practice theories, models, and methods—or combinations thereof—that best fit the client's unique circumstances and needs.

AMS is a perspective or framework for understanding clients. It relies on the practitioner's ability to use a variety of theories, models, and methods in their routine approach with clients. For example, an AMS practitioner will have the skills to apply different approaches to individual treatment (client-centered, cognitive-behavioral, etc.), family treatment (structural, narrative, Bowenian, etc.), work with couples, in groups, arrange for specialized care if needed, and, as an advocate on behalf of their client.

Practitioners must also know how to determine, primarily through the early engagement and assessment process, which theory, model, or approach (direct or indirect, for example) would work best for each client. Hence, successful practice using AMS relies heavily on the practitioner's ability to competently engage and assess client problems and strengths. Practitioners develop a sense of their client's personal interaction and relationship style—especially related to how they relate to authority figures—when determining which approach would best suit their circumstance. For example, a reserved, quiet, or thoughtful client or someone who lacks assertiveness may not be well served by a directive, confrontational approach, regardless of the practitioner's preference. Elsewhere we provide a more detailed exploration of the AMS perspective (Johnson & Grant, 2006, 2007).

DIMENSIONS OF AMS ASSESSMENT

To operationalize AMS from a client data collection and assessment perspective, below is a list, with brief explanations, of the dimensions of information needed. Collecting client information according to the following dimensions will provide the multiple systems data needed to develop a systemic understanding of each client.

A. Dimension 1: Client Description, Presenting Problem, and Referral

Beyond a physical and demographic description of clients, it is important to understand, from the client's perspective, what is/are the problems leading to the first session. Do not focus only on the problems that referral sources claim but learn the client's idea of the presenting problem. This may be anything from a recent arrest, to a drinking problem, to wanting to curry favor with a judge, or to get their family off their back. Whatever the client says is the problem is the problem you must address first.

A good practitioner also should understand how a referral was made, when, and the reasons. If it's a mandated referral (i.e., court, PO, etc.), it is helpful to discover the client's reaction to the referral. It is also important to explore the events or circumstances that led to the referral at this moment in time.

B. Dimension 2: Treatment/Therapy History

Include in this discussion any type of therapy, counseling, education, or more intensive treatments, inclusive of any problem. That is, explore past treatments for substance use, mental health, and others for the client and family members.

More than a place to record dates, places, and lengths of stay, this conversation should be targeted at what clients "thought" about their experiences. What did they like and dislike about treatment, therapists, counselors and/or programs, and their reasoning behind their beliefs? Also ask new clients about their expectations of therapy and therapists. An experienced clinician can use this conversation to learn a lot about how best to engage new clients, based entirely on their report of past treatment experiences.

C. Dimension 3: Substance Use History

Given the prevalence of co-occurring disorders across the practice spectrum, it is important for practitioners to gather substance use information about their client and his/her/their family, regardless of the client's presenting problem and/or the specialty of the organization. In this discussion, focus on age of first use of alcohol and other drugs for "recreation," substances used in the previous 30 days (including prescribed drugs), their favorite substances used in what combinations. Pay careful attention to the substances that clients mix together, hoping to understand if the combination of substances can lead to an accidental overdose.

If there is evidence of regular and patterned substance use, it is also important to discover if clients (or their family members) have ever been diagnosed with a substance use disorder. Understanding the role substance use, as a co-occurring disorder, can have on other problems, experienced practitioners would not perform any assessment without having explored the possibility substance use issues exist.

D. Dimension 4: Mental Health History

Data collected in this dimension focuses on symptoms, behaviors, thoughts, and feelings regarding both mental health functioning and potential mental health disorders. Practitioners can use one of the many mental health screening instruments available, including instruments designed to understand exposure to traumatic events and experiences. If there is evidence of trauma exposure, here is where practitioners explore the occurrence of events or activities leading to trauma reactions in clients. Explore past or present evidence of abuse and neglect (sexual, physical, emotional, domestic), exposure to violence, or being the victim of violence.

It is also important to learn about suicidal thoughts and gestures in the past or present, tendencies toward violence against family, strangers, etc., and other kinds of physicality that can stem from issues of mental health. It is also important to help understand the connections, if any, to the reports of mental problems and their substance use history above.

E. Dimension 5: Family History

Taking a family history helps place your client and his/her/their problems in the context of their family, defined as anybody your client considers "family." The most effective family history is one that comprises a look at three generations from the client presenting for therapy. Beyond the details of who is living, married, divorced, or deceased, explore the quality of relationships, problems across members and generations, and the level of support clients believe they receive from their families.

Experience teaches that problems tend to "run" in families, across subsystems and generations. A three-generation genogram with problems noted on the genogram provides clinicians with a quick and comprehensive look across the family that often helps explain your client in different ways. Practitioners cannot collect "too much" family history and background.

F. Dimension 6: Social Support and Engagement

In this dimension, explore with clients their social connections and the value clients place on these connections. The overarching question to answer here is, "When your life hits the skids, whom do you call for support?" Clinicians look to assess the degree to which people are connected to their community in productive ways, or disconnected, isolated, and/or alone.

Explore with clients support group attendance, social clubs, friends, family, and other groups they may be involved in, now and in the past. If they have quit these connections, discover their reasons for quitting. Also include their membership at places of worship, military history, workplaces, and/or any other group or people whom your clients find supportive. In addition, ask about your client's hobbies and what they like to do for fun. Have their interests narrowed over the years? Often, as problems become serious, people abandon activities, groups, and people, making their life narrow, losing the opportunity for positive social support (Johnson, 2004).

Do not ignore the supportive nature of engagements often deemed negative and counterproductive, like street gangs. These groups exist because they provide disaffected people with a sense of purpose, connection, structure, rules, and meaning. That is, street gangs and these groups exist largely because its members cannot or do not find these important and meaningful connections in their families and communities. Involvement in these groups demonstrates how important meaningful social connections are to people.

G. Dimension 7: Culture

While we provide a more extensive discussion of culture in practice later as a Guiding Practice Principle, it is important to inquire about client's cultural values, beyond race, gender, ethnicity, sexual preferences, and faith traditions. Culture represents more than demographics. That is, how do your client's cultural values shape choices, behaviors, values, and meaning (Johnson, 2000)? Practitioners must be aware that one's culture presents a fertile area for relying on stereotypes and personal bias. Understanding a client's culture has more to do with the ability to gather personal information from diverse clients than on a basic understanding of larger cultural groups and their tendencies. We are not concerned about how "Mexican families" operate, but about how the Mexican family in your office, right in front of you, operates and believes (Johnson, 2004).

H. Dimension 8: Biopsychosocial Connection

Helping students understand the impact of the biopsychosocial connection in clinical practice can be difficult. Certainly, in addition to the external effects of multiple systems on people, there is also the person as system to consider. After many years of trying different ways of explaining the biopsychosocial connection unsuccessfully, I heard the following explanation that makes the relationship clear.

For those readers sensitive to the use of the following analogy, I apologize. However, students have suggested this analogy makes the biopsychosocial interaction clear.

1. A person's biological dimension (including genetics), **loads the weapon**;
2. A person psychology (personality, coping mechanisms, attitude, etc.), **aims the weapon;** and
3. A person's social environment (friends, family, support, etc.), **pulls the trigger.**

Again, I apologize for the use of weapons as an analogy in a text like this, but if you think about it, it provides an apt description of how these three dimensions work together. Ironically, treatment, especially with clients experiencing co-occurring disorders, often works in the opposite order. That is:

1. Help clients create a supportive and helpful social environment to stop problem behaviors, or to stop pulling the trigger (i.e., substance use, mental health symptoms, ignoring medications, fighting, etc.);
2. Once the behavior has changed or ceased (periods of sobriety, calm, fewer symptoms, etc.), we can begin working on the person's aim toward problems or psychology involved by teaching new coping skills, relapse prevention, anger management, etc., through therapy;
3. Our profession does not have the technology, other than perhaps through medication, to change people's biological or genetic makeup.

Staying with the above analogy, while it is not today possible to "unload the weapon," it is possible to help clients stop "pulling the trigger" on problematic behaviors through social support, long enough to work on the underlying issues in therapy to change how people "aim the weapon."

In addition, several elements comprise the biopsychosocial perspective. Longres (2000) identifies two dimensions of individual functioning, the biophysical and the psychological, subdividing the psychological into three subdimensions: the cognitive, affective, and behavioral. Elsewhere, we added the spiritual/existential dimension to this conception (Johnson & Grant, 2006). Understanding how the biological, psychological, spiritual and existential, and social environment interacts is instrumental in developing an appreciation of how their environment influences individuals' influence.

GUIDING PRACTICE PRINCIPLES

AMS is based on several Guiding Practice-Tested Principles (GPP), derived from the current professional practice literature and the editors' 70-plus years of combined practice experience. The Guiding Practice Principles are the core—the guts, as it were—of the Advanced Multiple Systems (AMS) practice perspective.

Over the years, we have searched for the core of excellent practice. Hence, we developed the Guiding Practice Principles as the foundation of AMS as our way to approach this core. Here, Guiding Practice Principles (GPP) are defined as those precepts, ideas, attitudes, and practices used to guide an ethical, receptive, respectful, welcoming, and competent approach to clients and client problems regardless of the specific issues, culture, worldview, professional theories, models, or methods, professional disciplines, or practice settings. GPP describes fundamental ways of thinking and acting by human service professionals that, if consistent, transcend theory, model, or method. GPP is not tied to practice theory, model, or method; not bound by practitioner and client culture, practices, and beliefs. Practitioners may use any intervention or treatment choice to specifically match their client's culture or background, if that choice is deemed ethical and not in violation of one or more of the Guiding Practice Principles.

Like a professional code of ethics, the GPP are guidelines for thinking and decision making. GPP rarely describes specific rules or actions, but the larger goals of professional human interaction and relationship. Accordingly, as a practitioner, you can utilize whatever best practice or evidence-based theory and/or method deemed appropriate to help clients. GPP provides a helpful filter for practice decision making.

GUIDING PRACTICE PRINCIPLES EXPLAINED

First Principle (Umbrella Principle): Healthy Outcomes (and Lives) are Directly Related to People's Connections to Helpful, Supportive Systems, Across a Lifetime

The First Principle is universal ... it applies to everyone. That is, everyone who is either seeking a better life through therapy, counseling, and/or recovery or who lives a well-adjusted, healthy, and happy life abides at some level to the First Principle. Healthy people maintain lifelong, positive, and invariably intimate connections with helpful, healthy, and supportive systems throughout life.

We define helpful and supportive systems as any person, people, group, organization, program, etc., a person finds helpful and supportive; has the person's best interests at heart; and is one in which the person feels positively engaged. While the specifics and the nature of helpful and supportive systems change across a lifetime, the value of these connections is difficult to question (Johnson, 2004). They are the foundation of personal resilience. These relationships are the "difference that makes a difference" in treatment, recovery, life, and happiness.

Helpful and supportive systems also include counselors, therapists, and human service programs. But it is so much more in real life. Most people's "helpful and supportive systems" include everything from close friends and relatives to social clubs and groups, leagues, places of worship, coffee friends, support groups, etc. More importantly, a system is only helpful and supportive to the extent clients believe it is and **are willing to use it.**

It is not enough to say clients have "access" to helpful and supportive systems. We all have access to helpful and supportive systems. It does not matter that helpful and supportive systems are available—they are everywhere, personal, and professional. It only matters if a person is willing to seek and accept help and support from said system. Without personal investment and belief in its value as support, it is not helpful and supportive.

For example, it is only a partial step to give a client a list of Alcoholics Anonymous (AA) or Narcotics Anonymous (NA) meetings in the local area. Working to satisfy the tenets of the First Principle also includes discussing with clients what the organization is about, the reasons why it may be important for them to attend, the reasons why making friends and/or finding a sponsor is important. Based on your knowledge of the client, discussing with them before they attend what parts of the meetings your specific client may find difficult or objectionable as a way of removing excuses for not attending.

Why all this effort? Because we know attendance alone, without steps toward engagement in the process, will not provide long-term help and support. If you've heard the saying that people can be "lonely in a crowded stadium," then the importance of this discussion should be clear. One cannot be lonely in a crowded stadium, or an AA/NA meeting, if they are engaged with others and talking to people. To repeat—engagement, not access, is the key to successful social support in the First Practice Principle.

Hence, the First Practice Principle is the umbrella under which all else in professional practice falls. It is so important to understand and fundamental to long-term life success, and the **Final Practice Principle states: When all else fails, never do anything with and/or to a client that violates the First Principle.** Successful practitioners approach every client situation with the First Principle in mind, whether they know the specific definition or not.

What does this mean in practice? Those abiding by the First Practice Principle believe no matter how much or how little progress clients make, how resistant or unmotivated they may appear, or whether they do anything at all toward changing while in our care, they ensure clients do not leave their professional relationship angry, insulted, disillusioned, negatively labeled; or hostile toward help, helpers, and/or helping systems. At the very least, abiding by the First Practice Principle means helping set clients up for future success by not driving them away from care and/or helpers out of personal or professional frustration at the client's lack of engagement, motivation, or change.

The First Practice Principle requires both short- and long-term thinking. Is anything happening in therapy, or am I, as the practitioner, acting in such a way with my client today that may damage or make less likely he/she/they will be open to engaging with helpers and/or helping systems later in life when they might be more ready to change? In other words, how one is treated today will impact them in many important ways later. The First Practice Principle simply requires helpers to do everything within their power to ensure said impact is positive.

While we discuss client motivation later, it is important to understand the developmental nature of change and people's willingness to change. That is, people progress through different developmental stages related to the depth and severity of their problems, acceptance of their problems, the need for change, the motivation to change, and the courage and willingness to embark on a difficult and sometimes painful process called change (Johnson, 2004). Some make it; some do well and disappear, finding success through other services or support; some do well in the short term only to fade away; and, unfortunately, some never make progress and/or regress.

Often, when client progress lags, stalls, or never begins, often out of frustration, therapists often directly and personally confront clients about their lack of progress, engagement, or motivation with rude, accusatory, or even personally hostile remarks (Johnson & Grant, 2005).

The epitome of frustration occurs when therapists or counselors talk to clients, beginning with the phrase, "What you need to do is …" When I hear students or practitioners talking to clients in this way, I simply ask them, "Who in your life has the right to talk to you in that way?" Rarely do they have an answer. This approach is usually born out of the practitioner's need to control or be paternalistic, thinking of troubled clients more as children than struggling people.

In the substance use field, programs and practitioners often expel clients from treatment because they are not "ready" for change or because they experienced a relapse. At this moment, as you read this, all over the substance use treatment world clients are being dismissed from treatment for lack of progress; sent back out to drink and/or use drugs, risking arrest, injury, death, or the death of others so they can "hit bottom" and prove to the program they are "bad enough" or "desperate enough" to deserve help. The net result of these frustration-born tactics is to drive clients away from you, your agency, and perhaps the helping profession in the future. Why would someone ever want to seek therapy again after being treated in these ways? They probably would not.

In service of the First Practice Principle, our job is to ensure, as much as possible, when clients fade away from treatment or never get started at all, they do so based on personal choice and not because we "drove" them away through unusual behavioral expectations, attitude, inappropriate professional labels, misguided confrontation, attempts at control, and/or our professional or personal frustrations at their lack of progress.

Given the First Principle requirement of lifelong connections, it is good for practitioners to realize they are only a small part of the larger network of possible helpful systems a person needs during their lifetime. Unfortunately, we in the helping professions often see ourselves as far more, sometimes to the detriment of clients needing to establish their own personal networks.

Yet, while our professional role(s) is often short on the time line of lifelong connections, it can be the most important step in the process if we see to it clients make, foster, and utilize these connections during and after their time with us. That is, professional helpers play a seminal role in First Practice Principle work, largely because we become a client's initial "helpful" system. We are often the gatekeeper for help and lifelong change. How we interact with and treat people at perhaps the most vulnerable moment in their lives often determines the extent to which they will want to pursue other helpful systems in their lives in the future.

Hence, if we learn to treat even the most reluctant, angry, or resistant client with dignity, respect, and compassion, it is possible they may readily engage with us later, their next therapist or program, and/or find helpful and supportive systems in their communities. Not because the next therapist or program is necessarily "better" or "more skilled," but because your relationship formed the groundwork for clients to move developmentally closer to being ready for the excruciating work of changing their lives. Working to abide by the First Practice Principle may be more important in the long run than it is in terms of positive short-term, therapeutic outcomes. The First Principle is for life, not short-term gain.

The First Practice Principle consists of two important elements, each speaking to different aspects of the Principle. Indeed, it speaks to the importance of client engagement and the value of hope in people's lives.

Client Engagement

Fundamental to the First Practice Principle is the ability to rapidly develop rapport leading to client engagement. In this text, client engagement

> ... occurs when you develop a trusting and open professional relationship that promotes hope and presents viable prospects for change. Successful engagement occurs when you create a social context in which vulnerable people (who often hold jaded attitudes toward helping professionals) can share their innermost feelings, as well as [their] most embarrassing and shameful behavior with you, a total stranger, over a relative short period. (Johnson, 2004, p. 93)

Successful practice, regardless of setting or problems, is built on the foundation of trusting, respectful, and emotionally intimate relationships with their clients (Johnson, 2004). Clinical models and/or interventions are not effective without successful client engagement. Clients have no reason to accept help at a personal level from a therapist if they do not first like, and then come to trust and respect, them.

For example, I ask students to ponder how vulnerable, truthful, and motivated they would be with a therapist they did not like or come to trust and respect; would they accept help from anyone they did not trust or who did not treat them with dignity and respect? This is fundamental human relationship dynamics. To new clients, we are total strangers. They have no reason to trust or respect us when we meet. Simply having a college degree or an office with a "shingle" or because a judge ordered them to see us does not change basic, fundamental human relationship dynamics.

Becoming skilled in the nuances of successful client engagement is based on the fundamentals of being genuine, available, and focused on their clients. Most importantly, it is based on being friendly, open, welcoming, and polite, exhibiting these behaviors even when clients are hostile, angry, and resistant. When practitioners are nice and friendly, clients are not angry with them personally, but their own personal circumstances that led them to therapy.

Successful client engagement comes through understanding and accepting people's perceptions of their reality and not the "objective" reality of the practitioner. Seeking to understand how people perceive their world, problems, and the people around them increases the likelihood they will feel understood. This approach contributes to a professional relationship, based on the client's life and belief systems, is consistent with their worldview, and one that is culturally appropriate.

In short, understanding people's perceptions leads practitioners to understand each individual client's definition of "common sense." It is important to remember that "common sense" is only common and sensible to one person. There is no general definition of common sense. Common sense does not exist outside of people's social, environmental, family, and cultural contexts. It is unique to every person, depending on where they live and come from.

Being mindful of the definitions people learn from their culture underlies not only what they do but also what they perceive, feel, and think. This knowledge places practitioners on the correct path to "start where the client is." It emphasizes the cultural uniqueness of each client and the need to understand each client in their own context and belief systems, not the practitioner's context or belief systems.

Different people attribute different meaning to the same events, even within the same family or community. One cannot assume people raised in the same family will define their social world similarly. For example, the sound of gunfire in the middle of the night may be frightening or normal, depending upon where a person resides and what is routine and accepted in their specific environment. Moreover, simply because some members of a family are unfazed by nightly gunfire does not mean others in the same family will not be traumatized by it.

Additionally, people use language differently based on established or evolving cultural beliefs. For example, alcohol consumption is defined as problematic depending upon how the concept of "alcohol problem" is socially constructed in specific environments. Clients from so-called drinking cultures may define drinking six alcoholic drinks daily as normal, while someone from a different cultural background may see this level of consumption as problematic. I once worked in Russia and found an issue that demonstrates this point explicitly. Colleagues in Russia stated rather emphatically that consuming one "bottle" (approximately a US pint) of vodka per day was acceptable and normal. People consuming more than one bottle per day were defined as having a drinking problem. The normal, one-bottle-per-day level of consumption in the United States would be considered by most as clear evidence of problem drinking.

It is worth repeating: upholding the First Practice Principle requires the ability to engage clients in open and trusting professional relationships. The skills needed to engage clients from different backgrounds and with different personal and cultural histories are what drives practice, which determines the difference between successful and unsuccessful practice. Advanced client engagement skills allow the practitioner to elicit in-depth, personal information in a dialogue between client and practitioner (Johnson, 2004), providing the foundation for strengths-based client empowerment leading to change.

Fostering, Building, or Rediscovering Hopes and Dreams

Early in my career, I learned a lesson so important it became a hallmark of my practice approach. It helps me effectively engage clients from all walks and ages, races, ethnicities, genders, with multiple problems; the motivated, unmotivated, mandated, and hostile alike. It centered my approach on client motivation, long before models and methods came along to help with this (which we will discuss later). What I learned is:

> *Clients do not seek help because of their problems. They seek help because they lost the hope of being able to solve their problems on their own (or in their own social networks).*

Accordingly, helping professionals are not only in the problem-solving business but also in the "hope" business. What ... not in the problem-solving business? When someone comes to us because they drink too much, isn't it our job to get them to drink less ... or quit drinking? That's problem solving ... right?

Well, yes and no. Of course, as practitioners we want to help people change by solving their problems. There is no doubt about this. This might be the reason most of us endeavor to join this profession in the first place, to help people with their problems. Yet, most clients, even those with significant levels of personal denial, already know they need to change something, even if they will not admit it. Often, they already know what must change; they simply are not ready to admit it to us, mainly because they are not ready to assume responsibility to change. If all we needed to do is encourage people to change and have them do it, this would be easy work. Unfortunately, that is not how it works.

Our success, or skill, is not telling someone who drinks too much they need to quit drinking. Almost anybody can figure that out. The real skill—or art—of practice is getting clients to act even when they initially do not want to change. That is, before solving problems, our main task is helping convince people, at the deepest level possible, that change is not only positive and desirable, but more importantly ... possible.

First, an experienced practitioner helps clients discover, perhaps for the first time, that change is possible. When clients learn they too can change—that a better life is not just for "other people"—they can become motivated to solve problems in the short term and maintain short-term changes over the course of their lifetime.

Being clear, problems get solved by models, methods, and interventions; this is true. However, here we speak of the groundwork needed before models, methods, and interventions can work. To accomplish this, we first discover people's sense of **hope**; hope for a better future, hope for change, and hope they can be effective change agents in their own lives. Here, hope is defined as a person's expectation for the possibility of a better tomorrow, a sense of the future that develops over time and is a function of interactions between people and their environments.

While there is little consensus in the professional literature about what hope is, whether it is innate to the human condition, and/or how it is experienced (Polgar, 2017; Snyder, 2002), all agree having hope provides a sense of optimism for the future. An optimism that leads people to believe the difficult and painful journey toward a better life might be worth it. That is, hope for better, hope for different, and/or hope that change is even possible ... and good. A sense of hope, as defined here, is the foundation of motivation to change. With it, change is worth a try. Without it, why bother?

Of course, for many people, the prospect of hope for a better tomorrow is difficult, if not impossible to imagine. Their lives and existence preclude them from having hope for anything except, perhaps, survival. Whether it be from poverty, pain, violence, trauma, discrimination/racism, war, or their overall social environment, we cannot assume our clients know what it means to have a sense of optimism for the future; they are often devoid of the ability to dream.

According to Polgar (2017), "Most, if not all, who avail themselves of social work services live under siege conditions" (p. 271). That is, most clients find themselves under such significant personal and environmental stress, perhaps feeling under attack by their world, they end up focusing only on existing. People living under siege seek survival. They are often unable to visualize or imagine a positive future or engage in the kind of reflection required to realize, develop, or enhance hope for their future. Hence, people living under environmental siege can, at best, experience hope as an expectation there may be a tomorrow, but certainly not a better one (Polgar, 2017).

There are many people who do not understand, or worse yet, cannot allow themselves to believe in the idea, that a better life is possible and attainable. Perhaps their circumstances disrupted the ability to hope and dream from the beginning, or it was stolen or extinguished at an early age and never restored. Without a sense of hope and the ability to dream, people will not undertake the effort to change their lives with the sense of determination and motivation often required.

Yet, the loss of hope is usually larger than an individual problem. It also suggests a loss of hope in the ability of their friends, family, and other support networks to help as well. As I say to my students and workshop audiences, a lack of problems is not what separates us from our clients. Usually, what separates us is the ability to call on people we trust and love when life gets difficult; people who will support, challenge, and comfort us. These support people will have our best interests at heart and help lead us away from difficulty toward something more positive. Many people coming for professional help do not have this buffer, what we believe constitutes resilience. In our practice, we define resilience as the quality of one's social support network and one's willingness to use it. The better the support network, the more resilient people become.

Moreover, it helps to understand that the process of asking for or accepting professional help, defines in many ways people's lack of, or loss of, hope. For some, needing outside help in their lives is to admit they do not have "what it takes" to solve their own problems. Asking outsiders to help can be an outright violation of their personal, family, or community cultural norms. That is, asking for help is akin to admitting failure or weakness and can lead to a sense of shame and humiliation. Without taking these issues—hope, humiliation, and cultural norms—as a starting point for practice, change will most likely not occur.

People come for services discouraged, sometimes lost, having either abandoned their hopes and dreams or never knowing hopes and dreams were possible. Understanding this is, in our view, the core of practice wisdom. That is, without hope, either rekindled or newly discovered, long-term change is out of reach. Without hope, the kind of positive, healing, and powerful therapeutic relationship that leads to change becomes difficult. Hence, a respectful and trusting therapeutic relationship is more important in promoting positive clinical outcomes than specific therapeutic models or interventions (Johnson & Grant, 2005; Johnson, 2004).

Principle A: Clients Are People, Too

The main point of this principle is simple, yet so often not practiced. "Clients are people, too" is not intended as being funny or cute, but serious. Practitioners who embody Principle A in their worldview and practice approach will find success with client engagement and relationship building. This principle is important, respectful, and offers clients a sense of dignity at what could be their most vulnerable moment. Principle A is an integral part of Principle B (Practice Privilege) discussed below, but it also makes sense on its own. The best way to earn a client's trust and respect is for practitioners to act in trustworthy and respectful ways. There really is no other way to accomplish this feat. Therefore, Principle A: Clients Are People, Too, is defined as:

> *Practitioners should never expect their clients to act in ways the practitioner would not act in similar circumstances and under similar pressures. In fact, practitioners should never expect clients to act in ways practitioners do not act presently, in their private lives.*

I must ask, have you ever been late for an appointment, or class when your lateness meant nothing more than you were late? You were not late because you were "resistant" to your instructor or acting out in some meaningful, subconscious way. You were late. Period. If so, then why in the helping profession do we put so much time and effort into defining why our clients are sometimes late for their appointments? Even if they are late to every session, perhaps given their life circumstances, it's a major accomplishment to get themselves to your office. Perhaps they do not have reliable transportation. I've had a client tell me that their "ride" wanted sexual favors in exchange for the ride and they refused, making them miss the session completely.

Are there times when lateness or absence is a sign of avoidance ... sure. But without an open discussion with your clients about it and simply jumping to the conclusion that they are late just to make you mad, it means you do not think your "clients are people, too." Sometimes, people have good reasons to be late or miss a session that have nothing to do with the therapist or the session. It just did not work that day.

While the lateness example is oversimplified, it makes the point of this principle. People coming for therapy, by definition, have problems they cannot solve on their own (see First Principle above). Depending on their problems and circumstances, they may be under heavy pressure and stress from substance use, mental health challenges, children, divorce, poverty, lack of transportation, violence, abuse, neglect, etc. These are all serious issue that compromise people's ability to respond, process, follow through, and live up to a behavior contract or therapy plan as we think they should as motivated clients. Moreover, our client's lives can be toppled by what may seem to us middle-class therapists as the "smallest" things. We can claim "poor coping skills," but the fact remains our clients are often dealing with more than we will ever know or understand. Given the severity and difficulty of some clients' lives, it is a miracle of coping they can even get up in the morning, let alone make every session on time and fulfill a therapy contract from day to day.

When a client struggles to live up to our standards, first ask yourself the question: how would I respond under the same circumstances? This is called developing empathy. Have I ever not followed through on a work task? Have I ever been unfocused because of troubles in my personal life? Have I ever left my home a mess because I was too tired to clean it up? Have I ever been short-tempered with my partner, spouse, kids because of my stress and not because of them? Have I ever slept late, been late, skipped, taken a day off just because I felt like it instead of "being a responsible adult?"

If the answer is "yes" to any of these questions, then why is it "something deeper" when our clients do the same things? Give your clients the same benefit of the doubt we expect from others and ourselves, have empathy for people trying to navigate life. Discuss it with them, find out what happens to cause them to not follow through, and most of all, be open to cutting them some slack. After all, clients are people, too!

Principle B: Check Your Practice/Professional Privilege at the Door

Social privilege is a special, unearned advantage or entitlement, used to one's own benefit or to the detriment of others; often, the groups that benefit from it are unaware of it. It provides unearned access to resources that are only available to some people because of their social group membership, with immunity granted to or enjoyed by one group above and beyond the common advantage of others (www.ncjj.org/what-privilege, 2019). The idea of identifying the social privileges of certain groups (i.e., rich, white males) is an important conversation related to inequities and social justice. Social privilege is bestowed upon certain groups in certain situations by the larger system of forces and history, over many years, often to the detriment of everyone not in in the privileged groups. Let us take a moment and explore how this occurs.

Structural and Historical Systems of Privilege and Oppression: Who Holds the Power?

Often embedded in laws, policies, and social institutions are oppressive influences such as racism, sexism, homophobia, and classism, to name a few. These structural issues play a significant role in the lives of clients (through maltreatment, racism, and discrimination) and in clinical practice. How people are treated (or how they internalize the historical treatment of self, family, friends, and/or ancestors) shapes how they believe, think, and act in the present. Oppression, operationalized through privilege, affects how people perceive what others feel about them, how they view the world and their place in it, and how receptive they are to professional service providers. Therefore, culturally respectful and responsive practice must consider the impact of structural systems of oppression, social privilege, our practice privilege, and injustice on clients, their problems, strengths, and potential for change.

Oppression and privilege are by-products of socially constructed notions of power, privilege, control, and hierarchies of difference. As stated above, they are created and maintained by differences in power. Those who have power can force people to abide by the rules, standards, and actions the powerful deem worthwhile, mandatory, or acceptable. Those who hold power can enforce particular worldviews; deny equal access and opportunity to housing, employment, or health care; define right and wrong, normal and abnormal; and imprison, confine, and/or commit physical, emotional, or mental violence against the powerless (McLaren, 1995; Freire, 1993). Most importantly, power permits the holder to "set the very terms of power" (Appleby, 2001, p. 37). It defines the interaction between the oppressed and the oppressor, and between the practitioner and client. In the practice world, we as professional practitioners hold the power ... we have the privilege to enforce in our world in the same ways as dominant groups in the larger world.

Social institutions and practices are developed and maintained by the dominant culture to meet its needs and maintain its power. Everything and everybody are judged and classified accordingly. Even when the majority culture develops programs or engages in helping activities, these efforts will not include measures that threaten the dominant group's position at the top of the social hierarchy (Freire, 1993). For example, Kozol (1991) writes eloquently about how public schools fail by design, while Freire (1993) writes about how state welfare and private charity provide short-term assistance while ensuring that there are not enough resources to lift people permanently out of poverty.

Oppression and/or privilege are neither academic nor theoretical considerations; they are not faded relics of a bygone era. Racism did not end with the civil rights movement, and sexism was not eradicated by the feminist movement. Understanding how systems of oppression work in people's lives is of paramount importance for every individual and family seeking professional help, including those who belong to the same race, gender, and class as the practitioner.

Systems of oppression ensure unequal access to resources for certain individuals, families, and communities. However, while all oppressed people are similar in that they lack the power to define their place in the social hierarchy, oppression based on race, gender, sexual orientation, class, and other social factors is expressed in a variety of ways. Learning about cultural nuances is important in client assessment, treatment planning, and treatment (Lum, 1999). According to Pinderhughes (1989), there is no such thing as culture-free service delivery.

Cultural differences between clients and practitioners in terms of values, norms, beliefs, attitudes, lifestyles, and life opportunities affect every aspect of practice.

While larger social inequities are often discussed in terms of privilege, rarely have the helping professions examined and interrogated how professional or "Practice Privilege" operates in the relationships between practitioners and clients, clients and helping organizations, and how practitioners mediate the existing systems of oppression between clients and the larger social control systems (courts, CPS, mental health, etc.).

In the wrong hands, clinical training and practice bring the potential to exercise Practice Privilege to the detriment of our clients. Our professional degrees, licenses, certifications, and roles brings the power to define, label, and diagnose. We have the power to influence court decisions, parental custody decisions, existing relationships, and people's well-being. We make recommendations, give advice, judge, and decide our clients' futures and possibilities for change. In the wrong hands, we can dominate and define people's lives and the lives of their children well into the future, if not forever. This is the power of Practice Privilege.

This power is bestowed by the state and society as ours because we are members of this profession. We earn the right to be in our professional roles through education and training, but we do not earn the right to use it to shape and dominate other people's lives; to determine normal from abnormal, right from wrong, or healthy from unhealthy.

This notion of Practice Privilege must be considered, processed, and discussed in professional circles, much like the larger issues of social privilege. One of the insidious and consistent hallmarks of privilege is the people who have it do not know it exists, or when they exert it on others. This is difficult enough in daily life, but potentially harmful among professional practitioners.

Oblivious practitioners can wield Practice Privilege to the detriment of clients in professional practice without knowing it. Fighting one's privilege takes bringing the unknown to the fore, examining one's ideas and practices in a way that interrogates the extent to which our profession and our professionals wielding Practice Privilege that reinforce our client's place down the social hierarchy. Without a close, serious, and vulnerable exploration of our practices, much like we ask clients to do every day, we seriously cannot examine Practice Privilege, leaving us to blindly treat our clients in ways that reinforce their place and whose opinions and beliefs do not matter as much as those of the privileged few.

Principle C: Culturally Respectful and Responsive Client Engagement

Earlier, we defined client engagement as a mutual process occurring between clients and practitioners in a professional context created by practitioners. In other words, creating the professional space and open atmosphere that allows engagement to flourish is the primary responsibility of the practitioner, not the client.

Practitioners must have the skills and knowledge to adjust their approach toward specific clients and the client's cultural context and not vice versa. Clients do not adjust to us and our beliefs, values, and practices—we adjust to them. When that occurs, the foundation exists for client engagement. Relationships of this nature must be performed in a culturally welcoming and responsive manner. Yet, what does this mean?

Over the last two decades, social work and other helping professions have been concerned with cultural competence in practice (Fong, 2001). Beginning in the late 1970s the professional literature has been replete with ideas, definitions, and practice models designed to increase cultural awareness and promote culturally appropriate practice methods. Yet, despite the attention given to the issue, there remains confusion about how to define and teach culturally competent practice.

As stated earlier, over the years, many different ideas and definitions of what constitutes culturally competent practice have developed, as indicated by the growth of the professional literature since the late 1970s. To date, focus has primarily been placed in two areas: (1) the need for practitioners to be aware or their own cultural beliefs, ideas, and identities leading to cultural sensitivity; and (2) learning factual and descriptive information about various ethnic and racial groups based mostly on group-level survey data and analyses. Fong (2001) suggests that culture is often considered "tangential" to individual functioning and not central to the client's functioning (p. 5).

To address this issue, Fong (2001) builds on Lum's (1999) culturally competent practice model that focuses on four areas: (1) cultural awareness; (2) knowledge acquisition; (3) skill development; and (4) inductive learning. Besides inductive learning, Lum's model places focus mainly on practitioners in perpetual self-awareness, gaining knowledge about cultures, and skill building. While these are important ideas for cultural competence, Fong (2001) calls for a shift in thinking and practice, "to provide a culturally competent service focused solely on the client rather than the social worker and what he or she brings to the awareness of ethnicity" (p. 5). Fong (2001) suggests an "extension" (p. 6) of Lum's model by turning the focus of each of the four elements away from the practitioner toward the client. For example, cultural awareness changes from a practitioner focus to "the social worker's understanding and the identification of the critical cultural values important to the client system and to themselves" (p. 6). This change allows Fong (2001) to remain consistent with the stated definition of culturally competent practice, insisting that practitioners

> ... operating from an empowerment, strengths, and ecological framework, provide services, conduct assessments, and implement interventions that are reflective of the clients' cultural values and norms, congruent with their natural help-seeking behaviors, and inclusive of existing indigenous solutions. (p. 1)

While we agree with the idea that "to be culturally competent is to know the cultural values of the client system and to use them in planning and implementing services" (Fong, 2001, p. 6), we want to make this shift the main point of a culturally competent model of client engagement. That is, beyond what should or must occur, we believe that professional education and training must focus on the skills of culturally competent client engagement that are necessary to make this happen, a model that places the ability to gather individual client cultural information at the center of practice. We agree with Fong (2001) that having culturally sensitive or culturally aware practitioners is not nearly enough. Practitioner self-awareness and knowledge of different cultures do not constitute cultural competence. We strive to find a method for reaching this worthy goal.

Here, cultural competence does not mean practitioners will become competent in other people's cultures. This is not only impossible with limited exposure, but to assume it is possible is evidence of out-of-control practice privilege discussed earlier. We do not learn a "special" set of skills allowing us to transcend history, time, and our own culture to rapidly become competent in some else's culture.

Here, the central issue revolves around practitioners participating in inductive learning and the skills of grounded theory. In other words, regardless of practitioner beliefs, awareness, or sensitivities, cultural competence comes with the ability to gather the information necessary to understand their client's cultural values and meanings, and "ground" their theory of practice in the cultural context of their client. They develop a unique theory of human behavior based on the cultural beliefs and practices of each client. Culturally competent client engagement does not happen by assessing the extent to which client lives "fit" within existing theory and knowledge about reality, most of which is middle-class and Eurocentric at its core (Johnson, 2004). Cultural competence:

> ... <u>begins</u> with learning about different cultures, races, personal circumstances, and structural mechanisms of oppression. It <u>occurs</u> when practitioners master the interpersonal skills needed to move beyond general descriptions of a specific culture or race to learn specific individual, family, group, or community interpretations of culture, ethnicity, and race. The culturally competent practitioner knows that within each culture are individually interpreted and practiced thoughts, beliefs, and behaviors that may or may not be consistent with group-level information. That is, there is tremendous diversity within groups, as well as between them. Individuals are unique unto themselves, not simply interchangeable members of a specific culture, ethnicity, or race who naturally abide by the group-level norms often taught on graduate and undergraduate courses on human diversity. (Johnson, 2004, p. 105)

Culturally competent client engagement revolves around the practitioner's ability to create a relationship, through the professional use of self, based in true dialogue (Freire, 1993; Johnson, 2004). We define dialogue as "a joint endeavor, developed between people (in this case, practitioner and client) that move clients from their current state of hopelessness to a more hopeful, motivated position in their world (Johnson, 2004, p. 97). Elsewhere (Johnson, 2004), we detailed a model of culturally competent engagement based on Freire's (1993) definitions of oppression, communication, dialogue, practitioner self-work, and the ability to exhibit worldview respect, hope, humility, trust, and empathy.

To investigate culture in a competent manner is to take a comprehensive look into people's worldview—to discover what they believe about the world and their place in it. It goes beyond race and ethnicity (although these are important issues) into how culture determines thoughts, feelings, and behaviors in daily life. This includes what culture says about people's problems, culturally appropriate strengths and resources, the impact of gender on these issues, and what it means to seek professional help (Leigh, 1998).

The larger questions to be answered are how clients uniquely and individually interpret their culture; how their beliefs, attitudes, and behaviors are shaped by that interpretation; and how these cultural beliefs and practices affect daily life and determine lifestyle in the context of the larger community. Additionally, based on their cultural membership, beliefs, and practices, practitioners need to discover the potential and real barriers faced by clients in the world. For many clients of color and other minority groups, their worlds are defined by the racism, sexism, homophobia, and ethnocentrism that enforce limitations and barriers that others do not face.

What is the value of culturally competent client engagement? Helping clients discuss their attitudes, beliefs, and behaviors in the context of their culture—including their religious or spiritual belief systems—offers valuable information about their worldview, sense of social and spiritual connection, and/or practical involvement in their social world. Moreover, establishing connections between their unique interpretation of their culture and their daily life provides vital clues about people's belief systems, attitudes, expectations (social construction of reality), and explanation of behaviors that cannot be understood outside the context of their socially constructed interpretation of culture.

Principle D: Motivation Matters

Earlier, we discussed the importance of assessing a client's hopes and dreams for a better future as setting the stage for change. This, along with building a trusting, respectful, and culturally appropriate therapeutic relationship, all serves to enhance and bolster the client's motivation to change. Without the proper motivation, comprised of all we have discussed to this point, clients will continue to lack progress and/or success in therapy.

> *Remember our core belief: Clients do not change because of models, methods, or interventions alone. They change because they are helped into a trusting and respectful therapeutic relationship based on enhancing their dignity as human beings, have hope they can change for the better, and the motivation to endure the process of change. All of this is accomplished in the context of helpful and supportive systems of support to build personal resilience.*

Here, we look at ways to accurately assess your client's motivation for change. Miller and Rollnick (2002) suggest that clients with different stages of motivation, or change, require helpers to approach them differently, depending on the needs of their current stage of change and the needs to progress from earlier to later stages along the motivation continuum. The authors further state that "problems of clients being unmotivated or resistant occur when a counselor is using strategies inappropriate for a client's current stage of change" (Miller & Rollnick, 2002, p. 16).

In the 1980s, Prochaska and DiClemente (1982, 1984, 1986; DiClemente & Prochaska, 1985) developed the trans-theoretical model, commonly known as the Stages of Change model, based on their work with people trying to quit smoking. This model is based on how and why clients—either alone or with help—succeed at changing their addictive behavior. Subsequently, the Stages of Change model has been adapted for other addictive behaviors such as food and alcohol and other drugs (Connors, Donovan, & DiClemente, 2001; DiClemente & Hughes, 1990; DiClemente, 1991). Previously, we expanded the stages of change to include mental health disorders, trauma disorders, and other disorders (Johnson, 2004).

There are six stages of change to be assessed during an assessment and treatment process. It is important to note, however, the stages are fluid, meaning clients move from one to another, often needing between four and six "trips" through the stages before discovering long-term change (Miller & Rollnick, 1991). The stages of change are 1) Precontemplation; 2) Contemplation; 3) Preparation; 4) Action; 5) Maintenance; and 6) Relapse. The client's stage of change is assessed and determined for each diagnosable and treatable problem during each session. That is, if your client has two diagnosed co-occurring disorders (substance use and mental health), they are assessed along the stage of change continuum for each problem, during each session. These are described, along with assessment indicators, below.

1. Precontemplation

In the precontemplation stage, people have not yet considered the possibility they have a problem(s) or refuse to consider the possibility they may have a problem(s). Most often, clients in the precontemplation stage present with what appears as classic denial. These clients are often labeled resistant, recalcitrant, unmotivated, or not ready for treatment. They often refuse or make it difficult to perform an assessment, because they either have not considered their behavior as problematic or refuse to entertain a discussion about it. These clients are often mandated by outside systems, including the legal system, employers, or their families, but not always. Rarely will people in the precontemplation stage voluntarily submit themselves for treatment of any kind.

DiClemente (1991) suggests four subtypes of clients in the precontemplation stage. Called the "four R's" (DiClemente, 1991, p. 192), they include reluctance, rebellion, resignation, and rationalizing pre-contemplating clients.

Certain clients will fit the category of **reluctant pre-contemplators**. People in this category genuinely do not know or understand they have a problem(s) or even need to consider changing. These individuals are not as resistant as they are reluctant. Clients in this category will appear genuinely surprised, baffled, or taken aback by the suggestion they may have issues of any kind. They will appear as if they have never considered the possibility despite problematic behavior and significant negative life consequences. These clients require education and connections; problems and negative life consequences to their substance use and/or mental health disorders.

The **rebellious pre-contemplator** is resistant—resistant to being told what to do, to having their problems pointed out to them, and to most anything you do, except agree with them. If clients argue with nearly every question, refuse to respond or respond only in a hostile manner, and/or exhibit other oppositional behavior, it is quite possible you have a rebellious pre-contemplator in your presence. The best way to approach these individuals is to offer choices and/or to give the appearance you are not really trying to change them or "telling them what to do."

Resigned pre-contemplators have usually given up on the prospect for change and appear overwhelmed by their problems. Often, these individuals will want to tell you how many times they have tried and failed to quit, how nothing seems to work, and/or how they may be "destined" to be a drug addict. These clients lack hope. Throughout your conversation, they make it known it is too late for them.

Finally, **rationalizing pre-contemplators** have "all the answers" (p. 193). These individuals do not consider the possibility of change because they "have it all figured out." They know someone who has bigger problems, have plenty of reasons why their problem is not a problem, or believe they would be fine if people would simply leave them alone. Rationalizing pre-contemplators can sound a lot like rebellious pre-contemplators, with one exception, the rationalizing pre-contemplators will be intellectual, while rebellious pre-contemplators will be angry and emotional. If you begin to feel like you are in an intellectual debate with your client about the extent of their problems, she, he, or they are probably a rationalizing pre-contemplator. These clients need to be approached as such, asking them to explain how they came to their conclusions. Contradictions between what is said and what is happening in their lives must be pointed out and clarified.

2. Contemplation Stage

The contemplation stage is characterized by ambivalence (Miller & Rollnick, 2002). Clients in this stage are open to the possibility they have problems to work on and change may be needed. However, they have not yet decided to change and appear hesitant to make a commitment. This is a critical stage to recognize and one that can be quite frustrating, especially when you misread your client and act as if they are ready to change immediately. Miscalculations of this type often drive clients away or back into the precontemplation stage.

Clients in this stage will often state they know they should change and understand they have problems. They will give several reasons why they "should" change, but do not. The major difference is people in the contemplation stage acknowledge a vague problem exists and something "should" be done about it. To facilitate this ambivalence into a productive relationship, help clients explore past treatment failures, their fears about changing and staying the same, and offer hope that they can succeed. Clients in this stage, according to DiClemente (1991), lack a sense of self-efficacy needed to commit to a life changing process. In this case, not only is it our job to assess this stage, but to enhance it by employing approaches to help clients believe they have "what it takes" to succeed.

3. Preparation Stage

Clients in the preparation stage are already in the process of deciding to "stop a problem behavior or to initiate a positive behavior" (DiClemente, 1991, p. 197). These individuals have made a concrete decision to change. These are highly motivated individuals, ready to make a serious effort toward change. Clients in the preparation stage normally have already begun making changes or recently tried to change. They bring a serious commitment to their situation unseen in earlier stages. Your challenge is to enhance their motivation, offer support and linkages to resources needed to further their chances of success, and to discuss with them the potential barriers to change that may have to be confronted along the way. Helping clients through this anxiety and normal hesitation is critically important during this stage.

People in the preparation stage worry less about jargon, and more about what to do. How can you tell the difference between clients in the preparation stage and those who are not? Listen for reports about previous action, concrete plan development, and whether they have reasons for why they cannot begin the process immediately. In the context of the dilemma of change, people in the preparation stage will have misgivings, hesitancies, and fears about what they are trying to accomplish. They will not usually be adamant about the need to change, nor will they dismiss the notion that change is difficult and frightening. Therefore, if clients are adamant about the need to change and unwilling to address the dilemma of change, it is likely that they have not reached this stage.

4. Action Stage

People assessed to be in the action stage are committed to a course of action toward change (good or not). They have passed the point of decision making and are taking steps to change their life, perhaps attending AA or NA or therapy. If clients in the determination stage commit to and begin a plan of action (DiClemente, 1991; Prochaska and DiClemente, 1982, 1984, 1986), they move from that stage to the action stage. Hence, the action stage is characterized by your client implementing their plan.

5. Maintenance Stage

Occasionally clients will present in the maintenance stage, primarily for support. However, many of these clients find the support they need in community support groups (AA or NA), in their churches, synagogues, or mosques, or among family and friends in the community. The maintenance phase is the last stage of successful change. Over time, clients slowly replace old ineffective behaviors with new patterns. As the new behavior patterns, attitudes, and beliefs become firmly entrenched, old patterns dissipate. However, it is important to note that this takes time, perhaps years to accomplish. Clients who submit themselves for assessment at this point are usually trying to avoid and prevent a relapse, discussed next.

6. Relapse Stage

This is another stage where you will often find clients coming for assistance. They have cycled through the stages, often more than once, and achieved a period of maintenance through action. However, in any kind of treatment, relapse is a common and normal occurrence (Denning, 2000). For one reason or another, people often slip back into behaviors as they try to solidify their hold on their new lifestyle. These clients often come for assistance just after relapsing, with a weakened self-efficacy, guilt feelings, and a sense of resignation. The indicators of someone in the relapse stage are obvious. These are people who have been changing for any period who want to prevent a full-fledged relapse while continuing to make progress.

It is important to accurately identify your client's level of motivation by finding the current stage of change in which they exist during an assessment, for each diagnosed or treatable problem.

However, assessing his or her stage of change does not stop with the assessment. It is an ongoing part of the treatment process. Again, clients do not cycle smoothly through the stages, and relapse is a regular and expected occurrence in therapy, whether substance use or mental health. Also, remember that clients should be approached differently based on their motivation stage. For example, a client in the rebellious precontemplation stage cannot be approached harshly and directly. A more indirect approach that relies on slowly and gently pointing out discrepancies in his or her story is better.

Last Principle: When All Else Fails, Never Do Anything That Violates the First Principle!

This principle speaks for itself. If it will make your relationship oppositional, or if you are frustrated with your client's lack of progress, remember: Just. Don't. Do. It. In the end, if all else fails, practitioners can simply be nice, friendly, welcoming, and respectful. This attitude may just help save a life someday because they remember how nice you were when it comes time to seriously seek help.

SUMMARY

In this chapter we introduced you to the Advance Multiple Systems (AMS) practice perspective. This approach, although not a specific practice method, provides a foundation for conceptualizing and thinking about clients from a multiple systems perspective, particularly as it relates to understanding, engaging, assessing, and treatment planning for the cases included in this text.

We also exposed you to the Guiding Practice Principles of AMS. These principles, like a professional code of ethics, offer a process for clinical decision making throughout the treatment process. We place high value on the quality of relationships and solid personal choices always made in the client's best interest. We discussed the positive value of practitioners working to become the kind of professional who promotes trusting and respectful therapeutic relationships as the foundation for successful practice. We believe the best practitioners are personally insightful, attending to their personal biases, practice privilege, and relationships in a way that enhances their client's chance to succeed.

In the end, the following paragraph provides an excellent summary of the values and practices discussed in this chapter:

CORE BELIEFS

Clients do not change because of models, methods, or interventions alone. They change because they are helped into a trusting and respectful therapeutic relationship based on enhancing their dignity as human beings, have hope they can change for the better, and the motivation to endure the process of change. All of this is accomplished in the context of helpful and supportive systems of support to build personal resilience.

REFERENCES

Appleby, G. A. (2001). Dynamics of oppression and discrimination. In G. A. Appleby, E. Colon, & J. Hamilton (Eds.), *Diversity, oppression, and social functioning: Person-in-environment assessment and intervention.* Allyn & Bacon.

Connors, G. J., Donovan, D. M., & DiClemente, C. C. (2001). *Selecting and planning interventions: Substance abuse treatment and the stages of change.* Guilford Press.

Denning, P. (2000). *Practicing harm reduction psychotherapy: An alternative approach to addictions.* Guilford Press.

DiClemente, C. C. (1991). Motivational interviewing and the stages of change. In W. R. Miller & S. Rollnick (Eds.), *Motivational interviewing: Preparing people to change addictive behavior* (pp. 191–202). Guilford Press.

DiClemente, C. C., & Hughes, S. O. (1990). Stages of change profiles in outpatient alcoholism treatment. *Journal of Substance Abuse, 2,* 217–235.

DiClemente, C. C., & Prochaska, J. O. (1985). Processes and stages of change: Coping and competence in smoking behavior change. In S. Shiffman & T. A. Wills (Eds.), *Coping and substance abuse.* Academic Press.

Fong, R. (2001). Culturally competent social work practice: Past and present. In R. Fong & S. Furuto (Eds.), *Culturally competent practice: Skills, interventions, and evaluations.* Allyn and Bacon.

Freire, P. (1993). *Pedagogy of the oppressed.* Continuum.

Germain, C. B., & Gitterman, A. (1996). *The life model of social work practice* (2nd ed.). Columbia University Press.

Johnson, J. L. (2004). *Fundamentals of substance abuse practice.* Brooks/Cole.

Johnson, J. L. (2000). *Crossing borders—confronting history: Intercultural adjustment in a post-Cold War world.* University Press of America.

Johnson, J. L., & Grant, G. (2007). *Casebook: Sexual abuse.* Allyn & Bacon.

Johnson, J. L., & Grant, G. (2006). *Casebook: Mental health.* Allyn & Bacon.

Johnson, J. L., & Grant, G. (2005). *Casebook: Substance abuse.* Allyn & Bacon.

Kozol, J. (1991). *Savage inequalities: Children in America's schools.* Crown.

Leigh, J. W. (1998). *Communicating for cultural competence.* Allyn & Bacon.

Longres, J. F. (2000). *Human behavior in the social environment* (3rd ed.). F. E. Peacock.

Lum, D. (1999). *Culturally competent practice.* Brooks/Cole.

McLaren, P. (1995). *Critical pedagogy and predatory culture: Oppositional politics in a postmodern era.* Routledge.

Miller, W. R., & Rollnick, S. (2002). *Motivational interviewing: Preparing people to change addictive behavior* (2nd ed.). Guilford Press.

Miller, W. R., & Rollnick, S. (1991). *Motivational interviewing: Preparing people to change addictive behavior.* Guilford Press.

Mills, C. W. (1959). *The sociological imagination.* Oxford University Press.

Pinderhughes, E. (1989). *Understanding race, ethnicity, and power.* Free Press.

Polgar, A. T. (2017). Hope theory as social work treatment. In F. J. Turner (Ed.), *Social work treatment: Interlocking theoretical approaches* (6th ed.), pp. 222–275). Oxford University Press.

Prochaska, J. O., & DiClemente, C. C. (1986). Toward a comprehensive model of change. In W. R. Miller & N. Heather (Eds.), *Treating addictive behaviors: Processes of change* (pp. 3–27). Plenum Press.

Prochaska, J. O., & DiClemente, C. C. (1984). *The transtheoretical approach: Crossing traditional boundaries of therapy.* Dow Jones/Irwin.

Prochaska, J. O., & DiClemente, C. C. (1982). Transtheoretical therapy: Toward a more integrative model of change. *Psychotherapy: Theory, Research, and Practice, 19*, 276–288.

Snyder, C. R. (2002). Hope theory: Rainbows in the mind. *Psychological Inquiry, 13*(4), 249–275.

Timberlake, E. M., Farber, M. Z., & Sabatino, C.A. (2002). *The general method of social work practice: McMahon's generalist perspective* (4th ed.). Allyn and Bacon.

What is privilege? (2019). Online://www.njcc.org/what-privilege.

CHAPTER 2

Jeremiah Cartwright

Jerry L. Johnson

MY COLLEAGUE, RICHARD, referred Jeremiah Cartwright to me for outpatient substance abuse treatment after Richard said he could not engage him in therapy. According to Richard, he met with Jeremiah once, and they were "not a good fit." Richard made the referral because he thought my style would have a better chance of success with him. Since the early days of my career, I have worked on my ability to engage "difficult" clients. Even early in my career, what I lacked in clinical skill, I made up for by engaging difficult clients and keeping them in treatment. I've always enjoyed a challenge; I suppose this is a by-product of my early years as an athlete. Plus, I knew Richard would provide excellent supervision every step of the way. His support made tackling this challenge appealing. Jeremiah's case certainly qualified as challenging.

Let me explain.

JEREMIAH'S SITUATION AT REFERRAL

I knew little about Jeremiah Cartwright before our first meeting. I knew he was a 38-year-old African American male who was arrested for shooting at his wife of 11 years. Richard said Jeremiah awoke to a loud noise down the hallway from his bedroom, and "came up shooting" out of a deep sleep. Richard did not know how Jeremiah found a gun so quickly, or any other details because Jeremiah refused to speak about it with him. Jeremiah's twin toddler daughters were asleep in another room at the time but were not directly involved in the incident.

Fortunately, Jeremiah missed.

According to Richard, Jeremiah was previously arrested and convicted twice for drunken driving. He recently was arrested and convicted of Driving Under the Influence–Second Offense (DUI) 6 months prior to this event. He was on regular reporting probation for his second DUI. He had yet to be adjudicated for the shooting episode.

According to Richard, Jeremiah had a long history of drinking to intoxication. He also reminded me that Jeremiah's drinking and driving were especially problematic because he was a long-haul trucker.

It appears Jeremiah sought treatment at the behest of his attorney in hopes of limiting the punishment that was sure to come because of the shooting incident. Jeremiah's only interest, according to Richard, was to influence the judge. He had no other personal stake in seeking help.

QUESTIONS

1. Given what you know about Jeremiah and his current situation, what issues would you consider as you prepared to meet him for the first time?
2. Since client engagement seemed to be a problem for Richard, how would you prepare yourself to overcome the issues Richard described?
3. What are the most important factors in client engagement?
4. What percentage of your time do you spend working on and/or practicing your engagement skills? List several ways you can improve your practice engagement skills.
5. Before reading the next section, how do you approach involuntary clients in your practice?

WORKING WITH MANDATED CLIENTS

Jeremiah is what practitioners call an involuntary, mandated, or coerced client (Rooney, 1992). He sought help because of pressure or demand from the criminal justice system. He differed from so-called voluntary clients who choose to seek help. Jeremiah's only interest, at least initially, was to beat or mitigate the results of a pending court case.

Mandated or involuntary clients are a source of disdain for helping professionals because they can be difficult to treat (Rooney, 2002). That is, these clients do not begin therapy motivated to change. Often, they present as disinterested, bothered, and even hostile. Yet, often the problems of working with involuntary clients relate more to how practitioners define and approach so-called involuntary clients as opposed to those labeled as voluntary. That is, our approach, based on a predetermined set of behavioral expectations, can become a self-fulfilling prophecy. If we expect client resistance and hostility, we approach them as if it was sure to happen, often creating a relationship environment in which our attitude helps create the behavior we do not want.

In my experience, much of clinical practice education and training assumes clients are voluntary. That is, we often lead students to believe clients will answer questions honestly when asked and easily become motivated to change. We in the academy tend to assume most clients are ready, willing, and able to participate in their own treatment, and teach practice based on this premise. Little specific training or education is dedicated to the reality that practitioners will spend much of their professional career, especially early, in public agencies trying to treat involuntary clients mandated or coerced into treatment.

QUESTIONS

1. Think back over your educational career. What training or education have you received to specifically prepare you to work with involuntary or coerced clients?
2. What strategies have you learned or practiced that specifically address working with involuntary or coerced clients?
3. What is your attitude about clients involved with the legal system, and what factors contribute to this attitude? Where did this information come from: practice experience, personal bias, instructor bias, or some other place? Do coerced clients deserve the same consideration as other clients, or have they given up their rights because of their "offender" status? Search your attitudes and beliefs to uncover the possibility of negative implicit or explicit bias toward this population.

Over my 35 years in practice and education, I have seen few, if any, truly voluntary clients. While there are exceptions (people with the time and resources to pay for the privilege to understand their existential place in the world), most clients, even in private practice, seek help under some form of duress. They may come under pressure from an outside source such as friends, relatives, and/or employers or internal personal pressure after realizing their lives are not going well, or they are not happy or healthy, individually or in their relationships.

It is important to remember that even those who seek help from internal pressure often believe they "must" instead of "want" to seek therapy. It's the "must" part that often leads to engagement and motivation to change problems. In this way, self-referring or voluntary clients enter with a similar mindset as mandated clients who also "must" attend. The problem is not the clients, but the way practitioners think of and approach the two groups.

Therefore, it follows that most clients—regardless of practice setting or problems—will resist help and/or be resentful they need help, at least initially. Expect to find ambivalence to change, and do not mistake this ambivalence for client resistance.

I recommend practitioners consider client resistance or ambivalence (Miller & Rollnick, 2002; Connors, Donovan, & DiClemente, 2001) as a normal and expected part of the helping relationship, what I call the "dilemma of change" (Johnson, 2004, p. 124). The following passage exemplifies the dilemma of change (Johnson, 2004).

> Consider, if you will, the following definition: a dilemma occurs when a person is presented with two or more options, neither of which appears good. In this light, your client's hesitancy to change is understandable. Clients often say, "My life may be difficult now, but what if I go through all that work to change and my life is still miserable? At least now I'm high and don't worry about life much." This remark is not a function of resistance or denial, but an accurate appraisal of a real possibility. Clients are not eager to change, nor is it certain they will reap the benefits from achieving sobriety. In fact, many recovering substance abusers have said it took a significant period of abstinence, sometimes years, before their lives became better. For some, this improvement never happens. People do not change without pain (guilt, shame, embarrassment), struggle (multiple relapses), and/or without considering a permanent return to their previous life ("It wasn't *that* bad ... I had some great times on cocaine"). (pp. 124–125)

With Jeremiah, I approached him the same as I approach every client. I work to develop personal rapport (friendly, relaxed, social) while seeking to understand the context of the client's life, history, issues, and strengths as part of the process of establishing a relationship (Johnson, 2004). Early on, I do not challenge or confront directly, but ask challenging questions, listen, and try to understand. Any label (resistant client) that could cast the budding relationship in a negative direction (i.e., resistant client), has no place in early client engagement.

OUR FIRST MEETING

Jeremiah arrived 15 minutes late for his first individual session. Focusing on rapport-building, I presented myself as upbeat and encouraging while looking for a topic to ease our way into the session. Simple social conversation is a critical component of successful client engagement. My profession's title contains two words: social and work. Hence, there can be no "work" unless client contact begins with the "social" (Johnson, 2004).

In my practice, rapport relates to the early level of comfort clients feel with me, beginning with the initial telephone contact and proceeding through the initial conversation in the first moments of our meeting. Rapport can build quickly, but engagement takes longer. However, without rapport there can be no engagement.

I position myself so an already anxious and suspicious client can relax as quickly as possible. Accordingly, I did not mention his lateness for the session, but simply welcomed him in a friendly and casual manner.

Jeremiah was a thin, tall, African American man. He appeared tired and worn, as if he was living a difficult life. He appeared much older than his 38 years. He was casually dressed in relatively clean blue jeans and a button-down flannel shirt. He was wearing a tattered cowboy hat that he quickly removed upon entering my office. His cowboy boots were, however, beautiful.

Now, I'm not one to admire cowboy boots, but Jeremiah's boots were what I consider attractive footwear. They shined and glinted in my office lights. Almost the color of beach sand, they were adorned with what looked like hand-carved designs and some ornate stones mounted around the ankle and down the top of the foot bed. Clearly, Jeremiah liked his boots; and even more clearly, admiring his boots was a great place to begin our relationship.

"Man ... those are some nice boots you're wearing," I stated in an honest expression of admiration for his unusual footwear. "Where'd they come from?"

He looked down at his boots and extended his legs slightly in front of his chair so he could see them, almost as if he were looking at them for the first time. With a big smile and a hint of surprise in his eyes, he thanked me for noticing. "Not many folks like cowboy boots these days," he said. He explained he bought the boots while traveling over the road as a long-haul truck driver. They were made of snakeskin and hand tooled by a Native American artisan in South Dakota. The boots were Jeremiah's "pride and joy."

This exchange led to a conversation about his work. There was plenty of time to get to other issues later. In relationship building, it is important for client interviews to be unstructured. Working in an unstructured manner is how I operationalize the overused clinical practice phrase, "start where the client is." That is, once clients begin talking about themselves—regardless of what they talk about—I follow the conversation without overtly directing it. I never rush into so-called clinical issues. Everything clients say about themselves, including comments about cowboy boots, can be valuable in the engagement, assessment, and later, the treatment process (Johnson, 2004).

As it turned out, this seemingly casual conversation about cowboy boots and long-haul trucking was informative. I learned several important clues into Jeremiah's world that would prove helpful later. Had I not asked about his boots, I question when we would have gotten to this information in a way that made sense.

Jeremiah had been driving long-haul trucks as an independent contractor for 14 years. Truck driving was his only employment since his discharge from the military 15 years earlier. He said he enjoyed the "privacy and solitude" that came with his profession, and he made "excellent" money. When alone, out on the road, he was free from pressure and worry, alone with his thoughts and memories—free to try to relax. He craved the road and the sense of internal comfort it provided.

He worried about his wife and two children while he was gone, but also relished not having to be in the center of the "chaos" he said goes with being having twin four-year-old daughters. Most days, Jeremiah found it difficult to ease his worries, fears, and his sense of shame—what he calls his "traveling partners." Traveling alone over the road made his "partners" easier to manage.

The conversation segued from his internal "traveling partners" to his human life-partners. Jeremiah prided himself on being a family man. He married Fiona, a 35-year-old Iraqi-born woman 11 years earlier. He described their marriage as "good," citing the "normal" problems associated with marriage in general, with being in a cross-cultural marriage, and having young twins, specifically.

When asked what he meant, Jeremiah said both extended families raised serious objections to their marriage. While his family had come to grudgingly and distantly accept Fiona (his wife) as part of his family, his in-laws did not accept him. Their twin daughters were born four years earlier. He hoped having grandchildren would make Fiona's family "come around," but it had not.

Since he mentioned military service, I asked him about his service experience. Jeremiah served in the army during the second Iraq War, beginning in 2003. He enlisted out of high school and remained in the service on active duty through three tours.

When asked how it was to serve three terms in combat over a relatively short time, Jeremiah said it was "OK." He said he really had nothing to "rush home" for, and most of his duty was uneventful, until the end. It seems he had "pushed his luck," because his third tour was "different" from the previous two. While saying this, his body language and affect changed dramatically, from open and forthcoming to closed, dark, and flat.

Because this conversation occurred early in our first session, I decided to leave his life story there for a moment. I did not want to risk driving him away by pushing into intimate or painful territory before having the relationship basis for such a push. Pushing too hard or too quickly before a relationship develops often leads to inaccurate personal information and reduces the chance for a second interview. Despite my reluctance to proceed, his time in Iraq along with his emotional "traveling partners" seemed important. I was sure we would return to these topics if he decided to remain in therapy.

After thanking Jeremiah for saying a little about himself, I essentially "restarted" the session by discussing issues regarding informed consent. Clients who seek treatment under coercion or mandate need to understand and discuss the context of therapy in order to provide informed consent. I discussed with Jeremiah my role as a therapist, what would normally happen in a treatment setting with me, the limits of confidentiality, his right to refuse to speak or drop out of treatment at any time, and the potential consequences of this decision.

It can be difficult to discuss "housekeeping" issues without first briefly getting to know your client. This is the situation I was in with Jeremiah. The only information I had about him was the short history he provided during our cowboy boot discussion and what I had learned from Richard at referral. At the time, I still did not "know" about his drinking, the shooting, or the impending court case. This information came to me secondhand.

While it is appropriate to gather information about clients from referral sources, I rarely ask for too much information beyond the presenting issue and threat of harm potential. I never begin a session with information learned from referral sources. I want to hear about the client's life from the client. This allows me to be a learner and my client the teacher and sole informant about their life. Additionally, this approach limits my potential to develop preformed stereotypical "pictures" of clients based on personal biases or beliefs stemming from previous clients or my personal life-learning. The bottom line: I want to develop my own clinical impressions and professional relationship.

I encourage students and trainees to avoid the temptation to begin a first session with statements such as, "So, you were sent here because of your drinking?" This type of opening question is usually a sign that the practitioner is nervous, unsure of how to proceed, rude, or flat wrong. Jeremiah did not come to therapy for his drinking, he came to curry favor with the criminal justice system. Engagement works best when practitioners relax, help their clients relax, and proceed by having a "guided conversation" instead of a question-and-answer session—or worse yet, an interrogation.

The Shooting and Its Immediate Aftermath

"So, Jeremiah ... what brings you to see me today?"

"I really stepped in some shit this time," he responded, sighing while looking down at the floor. "I'm afraid I caught a serious case."

"You want to tell me about it?"

"I shot at my wife. I mean, I didn't hit her or anything ... I didn't mean it. She must have done something to startle me ... and I was having one of those nights. She knows better than to startle me at night."

With gentle probing, Jeremiah described the circumstances of the shooting. He claimed he had been sleeping, having one of his "restless" nights. At some point, his wife apparently opened and shut a door in the hallway outside the bedroom. The noise startled him awake. He remembers rolling off the bed, grabbing the handgun he kept between the mattress and box spring, and shooting in the direction of the noise. Jeremiah recalls hearing is his wife screaming at him to stop.

"It's almost like I was in a trance or something," he said, fighting back tears. It was clear this was traumatic for him and his wife, too, I'm sure. Among other things, shooting at his wife challenged his belief about being a proud family man.

"Then what happened?"

"The loud shot woke me up and I ran to her ... I couldn't believe what I did."

Jeremiah described his shock and horror at discovering he shot at his wife. He immediately called 911 and reported the incident. When the police arrived and learned Fiona was unhurt, Jeremiah confessed to police he was the shooter. After allowing them to arrange for a neighbor to watch his children, the police arrested Jeremiah for assault with a deadly weapon and aggravated domestic violence.

At his arraignment, Fiona pleaded with the judge and prosecutor to set low bail. Jeremiah was released on $5000 bail the next day.

After a long pause, I asked, "What did you mean when you said you were having one of those nights?"

From the look on his face (tense) and his body language (closed while turning away from me in his chair), this was a sensitive question.

"You know ... I was restless, having dreams about things. ..."

"Do you mind if I ask what you mean by "dreams about things?" I was being careful here not to push too far too fast.

"Yeah, I guess. Some nights I can't sleep ... I see things from Iraq and have dreams, you know. I remember things and that makes me restless and jumpy. I guess that was one of those nights."

He went on.

"Some nights I see those people, hear the noises, smell the smells, and feel like I'm back there in the shit. I don't know ... I just gotta get over it," he said with his voice trailing off, muffled by a deep sigh of resignation to the reality of his life haunted by the demons of war.

In the aftermath of the shooting, Child Protective Services (CPS) was enlisted to investigate Jeremiah and Fiona's ability to protect their children. The local CPS worker, in concert with the prosecutor and the police, elected to leave the two children at home with Fiona if Jeremiah agreed to move out at least temporarily until the legal situation was resolved and a custody decision could be investigated. In addition, Jeremiah had to turn over any and all firearms to the authorities.

Despite Fiona's pleadings, Jeremiah abided by the order and moved out of the house into a nearby hotel. He said he was relieved to move out for a while as he "couldn't bear to look his wife in the face" after what he "had done" to her.

Jeremiah's attorney recommended he seek professional help immediately. "So, my attorney gave me that other guy's name and he sent me to you. That's why I'm here."

Treatment History

"What happened when you met with Richard?"

I routinely spend time exploring a client's previous treatment experiences, trying to find clues about how to engage them in treatment (Johnson, 2004).

I am not as interested in dates, times, and lengths of stay as I am in the client's perception of their relationship with former practitioners, their likes and dislikes about the experience, and the client's perception and opinion about their former practitioner's "theory" of their problems. I always learn valuable information about how to approach and engage clients, and more importantly how not to approach certain clients.

"I just didn't like that guy," Jeremiah said. "It was nothing big, but I didn't like that he told me that I was an alcoholic and that I needed to take care of that first."

"When did he tell you this?"

"Damn … about 30 minutes after I met him. I didn't even know his name yet!" Jeremiah exclaimed. "I don't know why he said that. I came here cuz of the shooting … not cuz of my drinking."

The court had required Jeremiah to attend "drunken driving classes" on two different occasions following past arrests. He was unimpressed.

"They was a waste of my good time," he stated. "You know, lectures about the evils of drinking, and drinking and driving … and those movies with all the dead bodies. Hell, they didn't bother me, not with …" Jeremiah did not finish his sentence. "I just thought it was a waste."

He described his arrests for drunken driving as a combination of "bad luck" and "no big deal."

"Hell, as much as I drive, and I like to drink, I'm bound to get caught. It's no big deal. It certainly doesn't mean I'm a drunk!" He went further, "I got friends been arrested four or five times and they're not drunks … I guess I'm just livin' under a dark cloud."

"Is drinking something you don't want to talk about then?"

"Nah, we can talk about it all you want. I'm telling you that I don't have a drinking problem … I am not an alcoholic!"

Since I only knew Jeremiah at this point for about 30 minutes, his response to the last questions served as both a warning and provided valuable information. While he was willing to discuss shooting his wife, his war experience to a point, and drinking per se, he was not open to discussing the possibility of a drinking problem. The warning—if I pushed him, as Richard apparently had—he was leaving treatment. While leaving treatment is certainly his choice, I did not want it to happen because I was clumsy or in a hurry as a therapist. If he drops out, I want it to be his choice because the work is too difficult, not because I could not take a hint.

The important information was Jeremiah said we could talk about his drinking. In addition, he provided a lot more information about it and what drinking does for him than Richard learned. This was encouraging.

This is familiar territory for practitioners who work with substance abusing clients everywhere. Most clients are either unwilling to discuss their use or unwilling to tell the truth about their use even if they discuss it. Simply looking at what I thought I knew about Jeremiah's drinking (multiple drunken driving arrests, statements about his daily drinking, and his sensitivity toward the subject), it would have been easy to assume, based on my experience with others, that Jeremiah probably had a serious alcohol use disorder.

In my colleague Richard's defense, he worked from a disease/medical model promoted through Alcoholics Anonymous (AA) and other 12-step support groups and commonly used in treatment centers across the United States. From this perspective, Jeremiah must work solely on quitting drinking before working on any other issue, including possible co-occurring mental health disorders. This is usually approached with specific and direct personal confrontation of what appears to be client denial of their problems. There are still 12-step support groups today that believe taking prescribed medication for co-occurring mental health disorders constitutes a substance use relapse. So, Richard followed the disease model playbook. The only problem? It did not work with Jeremiah.

It was clear based on Jeremiah's anger at Richard that I would need a different approach in this case. That is not to say I am opposed to the disease model, because I am not. I am not loyal to any approach. I am more pragmatic, especially early in treatment. I still did not know him. I did not know if he had a drinking problem, despite the drunken driving arrests. I suppose it was possible that he was the unluckiest fellow in the world.

My interest, even if he had not warned me about the touchiness of the subject, was to understand Jeremiah Cartwright, not to assume he had a problem with alcohol use, and not tell him about it, <u>even if I thought he did</u>. It is possible Richard's assessment was correct, but certainly his approach and timing were poor. I always believe it is not what practitioners say that causes problems, but when and how they say it. Timing is everything.

"Why do you think Richard thought that you were an alcoholic?"

"I don't know," Jeremiah said in an excitable tone. "You tell me!"

Instead of answering his question, I asked more of my own. "Did he ask you a lot about your drinking?"

"Yeah … that's all he asked about. I drink, yes, sometimes a lot and most every day at that. Always have, but that's not a deal I can worry about now. Shit, man, I shot at my wife and might be going to prison."

Notice he said he could not worry about drinking "now." This was a revealing statement providing encouraging and potentially positive signs for later. Perhaps he had been wondering about his drinking as a problem after all. I guess timing is everything.

"Yeah, you could be going to prison, for sure. What do you hope coming to me can do about that possibility?"

"I don't know. My attorney thinks if I come to counseling it might help show the man I'm sorry and serious about not letting this ever happen again."

"And if he (the judge) thinks that …?"

"Then maybe I won't get any time for this. I mean … Fiona has forgiven me. She understands …"

"She understands what?"

"I didn't mean to. I'm not a violent man … I love my family … I've just been all confused lately. Some days it's worse than others."

"How long you been confused?"

"Since the war, man," he said while looking away, his voice trailing off. "I think the war might be messin' with my head. … I don't know …"

"Do you think drinking is part of your confusion?"

"NO! Hell, it's about all that helps."

We reached the end of our session. I had to move toward terminating the session and try to elicit his agreement to come back for a second session. In his case, and after the seriousness of the information we discussed, his return would be a positive indicator he was engaging in treatment.

"Jeremiah, I'd sure like to look at your confusion with you, if that'd be okay."

He nodded in apparent agreement.

"I don't know if I can help, but I can sure give it a try, if you're up for it. How about another meeting next week?"

"All right."

With that, we ended. I thanked him for coming and discussing his personal "business" with me, a total stranger. He sighed, which I interpreted as an acknowledgment the session had indeed been difficult. We scheduled for the following week at the same time. He left after a handshake. I wasn't sure if his departure was from this session, or treatment entirely. I hoped to see him again.

QUESTIONS

The author took a nonconfrontational approach, concerning himself more with engaging the client than getting his entire story. Yet, many substance abuse practitioners would believe a more direct approach is what clients with substance abuse problems need to help with their denial. This is more than simply a theoretical or style difference. The professional literature is now producing a body of research that specifically addresses this difference. Therefore,

1. Explore the substance abuse and treatment literature looking for evidence of the efficacy of both a nonconfrontational approach and a confrontational approach in substance abuse practice. Develop a position based on a balanced exploration of all sides of this argument.

At the end of the first session, Jeremiah revealed important clues about his problems, experiences, and worldview.
2. Based on the information given in the first session, generate a list of Jeremiah's problems and strengths.
3. What is your initial assessment? Write it down in a concise, one-paragraph narrative form as if you are writing an article abstract of this session.
4. What areas of Jeremiah's life need further exploration in the next session, and how do you plan to approach the issues when and if he returns?

SESSION TWO: ALCOHOL AND DRUGS

I was busy in the days leading up to Jeremiah's next scheduled appointment. Yet, I wondered all week whether he would return. Happily, when I walked to the small waiting area of our offices, there was Jeremiah sitting in the corner reading a sports magazine—10 minutes early! Dressed this week in what appeared to be the same clothing as before, he walked into my office and found his seat.

"It's good to see you," I said.

"Yeah ... I wasn't going to come back, but my wife said I really should. So, I'm here because of her."

This is another common response. Jeremiah would not admit to coming back on his own, so he blamed his wife. This was his way of saying, "I am not ready to admit that I want this, so I'll say I'm doing it for my wife." Maybe he was. We would find out soon, I was sure.

Since I tend to pay more attention to actions than words, especially when working with mandated, potential substance use disorder clients, Jeremiah's return for a second visit meant a relationship had begun. Notice I said "begun" and not "developed.' We were still a long way from having a "developed" therapeutic relationship.

I had two primary goals for this visit. The first was to collect as much life information as possible, hopefully focusing on his family, substance use, possible mental health challenges, military service, and the shooting. My second goal was to monitor our relationship in hopes of strengthening what we had started. The extent to which I accomplished the second goal would directly determine how we did on the first. Jeremiah would determine how deeply we dove into his life story. There will come a time when I will be firm, just not this early in treatment.

"How you been, Jeremiah?"

"It's hard, man. I hate that damned hotel, but I'm not ready to go home yet."

"Why not?"

"I'm ashamed ... Fiona wants me home, CPS said it's okay if I go home, but I'm still having trouble looking at her."

"What will have to happen before you can look at her again?"

"Time, man, I just need some time ... but if those idiots at the hotel keep partying all night, I might need less time that I thought," he said with a laugh. "I just gotta work some things out in my head."

"Such as?"

"You know ... some things. Like, how could I do this and how can I face her, that kind of shit. I'm the kind of guy that needs to think stuff through ... figure it out for myself before I talk about it."

Jeremiah just sent another "slow down" message. "Okay, I'd be happy to talk about that stuff when you're ready" I said, pausing in such a way that made changing the subject more natural and my intentions to do so obvious. My sense of the conversation and his body language (closed and rigid) led me toward a less threatening approach.

"I was hoping to learn more about you, your family and things like that. Sound all right with you?"

"Yeah, sure. What do you want to know?"

I like to build a three-generation genogram while taking family and personal history. A genogram is a graphical way to describe a person's life and issues in the context of their family system (Bowen, 1985). While I happen to use a genogram format, there are many ways to achieve the same result. It is important for practitioners to find a style, procedure, or format that allows them to collect system-based client information in a way that makes sense to the practitioner.

Whatever the format, try not to turn this important function into a question-and-answer interrogation. My advice: generate a conversation about your client's life and times. It is difficult to build a conversation around a series of preordained and preordered, close-ended questions. When clients start talking, they reveal more than when they are interrupted by rapid-fire questions.

"Let's start by talking about your family. If you don't mind, I will be drawing a picture of your family while we speak. I need pictures to remember," I said, laughing.

"Getting old is a bitch, huh?" Good. Jeremiah felt relaxed enough to joke with me.

Jeremiah's Extended Family

Jeremiah was the second of four children born to his biological parents, Fred and Betty. Fred and Betty married 41 years ago, prior to their moving north from Mississippi in search of work and a new start away from "the rednecks and bigots" in the South.

Jeremiah's father was a 67-year-old African American man, retired after 35 years working the production line for a major automaker. He described his father as a strict disciplinarian, who demanded his children stay out of trouble and follow orders. His father always said the way for Blacks to survive was to obey the law and keep quiet—never give the White man any reason to notice you. Of course, in Mississippi during the 1950s and 1960s, Whites did not need a reason to go after Blacks in the South. According to Jeremiah, their southern heritage and links to a slavery and Jim Crow past were important in his family, mostly because of his father's constant reminders.

Jeremiah's father took pride in supporting his family, often working overtime so his family could live well. His father always said, "No more sharecroppers in this family." Since his retirement, his father had been "hanging around the house," meeting friends to play cards and trying to enjoy life. He also said his father was a lifelong drinker, "nothing serious," but he had been drinking more since retirement. Jeremiah was careful to say his father was not an alcoholic. "He's a strong man who can handle his liquor … besides, after his life, he deserves to drink if he wants to."

I simply nodded and moved on.

At 67, his mother, Betty, was about to retire from her career as a schoolteacher. She returned to college and earned her teaching certificate some years ago, a proud moment for his father and the family. Jeremiah described his mother as a "woman of deep faith," who was the "heart and soul" of the family. Mother was the person who insisted the children attend church, do well in school, and graduate from college ("the best way to keep out from under the White man").

While Jeremiah said he loved and respected his father, his mother was the most important person in his life next to his wife, although they had become "distant" since he left for and returned from the war. Mother brought "balance" to their lives, while his father provided strictness, discipline, and a keen sense of family and cultural history. Jeremiah insists his mother remains "deeply disappointed" in his choices many years ago, although admittedly they have not discussed it in 20 years.

"We haven't never gotten over it."

Jeremiah described his older sister (40 years old) as a person with "problems." She had been married twice and had one child from her first marriage. That marriage dissolved when the family learned her husband was physically abusing her. Jeremiah described him as a "dope fiend" who could not control himself. He blamed her ex-husband for getting his sister into drinking and eventually, drug use. She recently remarried but, according to Jeremiah, the marriage was doomed. They were both heavy drinkers and drug users.

He did not worry about his nephew, because he mostly lived with Jeremiah's parents. Fred helped his sister get a job at the same plant as he, but the family worries she might get fired because of her drinking and other problems. "Losing her job would send her way over the edge," according to Jeremiah.

Jeremiah's younger siblings (sister, 32 years old, and brother, 30 years old) were both single and worked at the auto company. He said both siblings were "doing well" and neither had any significant problems. The youngest brother still lived in his parents' home. His sister lived locally and spent a lot of time with their parents.

Jeremiah was friendly yet distant from his younger siblings. However, he was so "pissed off" at his older sister he refused to speak to her. His anger, Jeremiah said, came from her drinking, drugs, and not taking care of her child.

"We were raised better than that," he exclaimed, oblivious to the irony of that statement given his current predicament.

"It looks like (the auto company) is a family tradition. How come you didn't follow your father's path?" I asked.

"I could have, if I wanted to. Even though times were tough, my father promised me a job on the line. He and Mom really wanted that for me. But … I didn't. I couldn't see being trapped on that line for the rest of my life. It's good for him and the others, but not for me. So I joined the army instead. The truth is, I really decided to enlist when 9-11 happened … really pissed me off."

"How'd your father take that decision?"

"Not good, not good at all. We're still not good behind it after all these years. I'm sure he's convinced the army and the war are why I have problems … and why I shot at Fiona. My father believes "the demons got hold of me … and he's probably right about that … but still, we aren't friendly at all."

"The bad part is that I'm not close to any of them anymore."

"What do you mean? Can you call them for help if you need it?"

"No. I don't know. I think they see me as the child who joined the White man in his wars … even my mother and I haven't really spoke in years … since the babies were born."

"What did your Dad mean by the demons?

"You know … the memories and fears, the stuff that comes from war." Jeremiah was almost whispering. Then, in a sudden change of attitude and affect, he uttered, "I don't want to talk about this shit … not now. What else you need to know?"

Fiona's Extended Family

Fiona is the elder of two children. She was born in Iraq as a Shia Muslim and moved to the United States with her parents when she was young, escaping the discrimination, repression, and retribution from Saddam Hussein, who was Sunni. According to Jeremiah, her parents were strict Shia Muslim Iraqis who believed in abiding by their culture.

Among other things, they believed Fiona should have married in her race and faith, not to an American and especially not an African American. They were also furious because Jeremiah was not a Muslim. To their consternation, Fiona moved away from her parents' faith tradition and married against their wishes.

According to Jeremiah, their marriage brought "great shame" onto Fiona's family here and abroad.

"Good thing they don't still do honor killings," Jeremiah chuckled, only partly joking.

Fiona's father owned and operated a small business in the city. He worked long hours for relatively little wage. Fiona's mother primarily cared for the family when not helping her husband in the family business, where she served as bookkeeper.

Her parents immigrated to the United States years earlier and found a growing Middle Eastern community in the metropolitan area, mostly Iranian in those days. In recent years, there was an influx of Iraqi refugees as well. According to Jeremiah, Fiona's parents maintained most of their traditional values, including language. The family spoke Arabic in their community and in Jeremiah's presence.

"That really bothers me. They won't even speak to me in English. I always feel like they're making fun of me. It's like I don't even exist to them."

Jeremiah and Fiona hoped the grandchildren would ease the tension, but they did not. While her parents "love" their grandchildren, they refuse to speak to Jeremiah and are constantly trying to "get Fiona to divorce him and come home to their faith and family."

"What do you think is happening since the shooting?" I asked.

"Wow ... I'm sure they're giving her some serious crap now."

"Has she said anything?"

"Nope, but she wouldn't. Fiona tries to keep this stuff away from me ... especially now, I'm sure."

Fiona's younger sister married an Iraqi man five years earlier. They had one child and live in the same community as her parents. Jeremiah's sister-in-law worked part-time in the family business, and his brother-in-law worked for a local computer company. While Jeremiah claimed Fiona's sister and husband were friendly people, there was tension. Fiona had a relationship with them, but kept it secret from her parents. According to Jeremiah, Fiona's sister had hoped Fiona would find a nice Iraqi American man to marry.

"Oh well, guess I don't qualify," Jeremiah said.

Jeremiah and Fiona

Jeremiah met Fiona after returning from his last tour of duty. They immediately began dating and were soon engaged. They married three years later (11 years earlier), despite the problems with both extended families. In fact, Fiona's family refused to attend the wedding. Jeremiah's father gave Fiona away in place of her father. Before the children were born, Fiona worked various jobs in retail. She liked working, but her heart was set on having a family. She often stayed with her sister during Jeremiah's many overnight trucking assignments.

Jeremiah described Fiona as a loving woman who understood him and what his life was like since the war. "She is the only one who understands me. And now I go and do this."

He described Fiona as an excellent mother, the person who held the family together when he was working or unable to be around because of his "traveling partners."

"She would do anything for us. I was really lucky to find her," he stated. "Plus," he said with a smile, "she's beautiful." He described Fiona as "a light-brown-skinned beauty ... thin, with long shiny and silky black hair. I love just looking at her."

Four years ago, Fiona gave birth to their first children—twin daughters. While Jeremiah was happy to have children, the additions caused problems. The chaos that came with children, especially to first-time parents, intensified because they had twins. While Fiona loved the added responsibility and the "constant noise," Jeremiah was troubled.

"I have a hard time with all the stuff that goes on ... all the time."

"What stuff?"

"You know, the noise, the crying, and the constant mess that goes with having two children at once. It makes me nervous and edgy ... I just want to get away from it. Sometimes, I just have to go ... I have a hell of a hard time relaxing."

He went on, clearly agitated, "Don't get me wrong—I love my kids. They are my babies and I would do anything for them and Fiona. I mean ... it's not them, it's me. Sometimes I can't take it."

"What do you do when it gets to you, Jeremiah?"

"I get out of the house. It's not that I get mad ... I don't get mad at the kids, don't hit them or anything like that. I just have to leave."

"Where do you go? Do you have friends that you see?"

"I don't have many friends. In fact, I don't think I have any friends. Since the war, I've not been the kind of guy to have buddies. I have my work, Fiona and the kids ... that's enough for one person. I like to be alone. It calms me down."

"Have you stayed in touch with childhood friends, or from the service?"

"Naw ... I bump into old high school friends from time to time, but I don't want nothing to do with dudes from the service. That's over for me ... done!"

"What else do you do to relax during these times?"

"I drive, I like to drive, either the truck or my car. Fiona knows this and she never gives me any shit about it. I just need to get away for a while, and then I'm fine."

We arrived at another important moment. The next logical question pertained to Jeremiah's drinking, since he loved to drive, drove for a living, needed help relaxing, and had multiple drunken driving arrests.

"Do you ever drink to help you relax?"

"Yeah, sometimes I do. Having a few takes the edge off, that's for sure."

Drinking and Legal History

That went well. I decided to keep pursuing this line of questioning and see where it took us.

"How long have you been drinking, Jeremiah?"

After hesitating, he said, "Since I was 12 or so ... had my first drinks at a family retirement party. My grandfather retired and I ran around drinking half-filled drinks left by everyone."

"How about now, do you drink regularly?"

"Yeah, I do. I drink something every day. I like how it tastes, but like I said, it takes the edge off. Makes me relax."

"Have you noticed a change in how much or how often you drink since the shooting?"

"I guess ... I'm drinking more in the last few weeks. I don't have the kids or Fiona around, and I haven't been working. So, I drink. It helps, man."

"When did you begin drinking regularly? How old were you?"

"Oh, probably 16—weekends, parties, football games ... you know, the high school shit."

"When did it become more than weekend party stuff?"

"I was drinking more before I enlisted, but it really began in Iraq. ..." His voice trailed off. "There wasn't much else to do over there 'cept drink. They wouldn't let us smoke weed."

"Still smoking weed (marijuana)?"

"Nope, that was one thing Fiona called a halt to. She didn't care if I drank, but no drugs ... and I haven't since we met."

As it turns out, my colleague was correct. Jeremiah had a long history of drinking to intoxication and legal troubles stemming from his drinking. I was not accusing him of having a drinking problem. He stated earlier he was willing to discuss drinking, just not drinking problems. Richardlin (1992) states that because of the long history of negative labeling by the white majority, African American men are sensitive to any labeling. They need to feel part of any labeling decision, including the decision about the nature and extent of their problems. That hurdle was yet to come.

Jeremiah said he graduated from casual social drinking during high school to regular, daily, and heavy drinking just before and during the war. Soon after arriving home from the war, both during his dwell time between tours and after he was discharged, he was drinking about 12 "beers" per day and a pint of liquor. Over the years since his discharge, his drinking remained at or near this average daily level.

He reported frequent alcohol-related blackouts and feared he would have physical withdrawal if he went without drinking for more than one day. He experienced the "shakes" every morning but warded them off with "a little something" in his coffee. He also said he tried to cut down several times, to no avail. The longest he went without alcohol since the war was two days, when he was in the hospital for knee surgery. That was five years ago.

Since the shooting, Jeremiah said his drinking increased "quite a bit." He went on to say he drank on the day of our meetings, just enough to be calm but not enough for it to show. He would drink as soon as he left my office. His current routine was to retreat to his rented hotel room with a case of beer and a bottle of gin, watch television, and "think."

Jeremiah said he smoked marijuana daily after his discharge for a couple of years. He had, however, not smoked weed or used any illegal drugs since he met and married Fiona.

Jeremiah also said he is not taking any prescribed medication for anxiety or depression, or any other mental health disorder. "I ain't crazy like that."

"What I got seems to work just fine," he said with a chuckle.

"Has drinking ever caused you any troubles—legally, personally, on the job—stuff like that?"

"Oh, yeah, it has. Not at home or with my family, but I seem to be somebody that gets caught drinking and driving."

He told me about his two arrests for drunken driving over a 10-year period, most recently within the past year. He was on probation when the shooting occurred. He said he never did any jail time for his convictions, always receiving probation and drunken driving school. His attorney, a specialist in drunken driving offenses, was able to keep him out of jail and keep his driver's license current because of Jeremiah's professional and family responsibilities. Jeremiah could not earn a living and support his family without his CDL (Commercial Driver's License).

On the day of the shooting, Jeremiah had been drinking "hard." He spent the day in front of the television watching football games. He claimed he had consumed "at least a case of beer," enjoying a "relaxing day of football." He fell asleep early, but was restless all night, disturbed by his dreams; dreams of the war and the people he once knew who were dead. Then he heard the door slam; he startled awake, and in a fog, shot at the noise. Unfortunately, he wasn't in Iraq, but in his bedroom. The noise wasn't the enemy; it was his wife, coming out of the bathroom.

We were nearing the end of a very painful and tiring session, but I had one more question for Jeremiah, one that could either make or break the remainder of our time together. I had to ask.

"Jeremiah, have you ever wondered if your drinking was a problem?"

There was a long pause, perhaps 20 seconds. It seemed like 20 minutes. Looking down and then up directly into my eyes, he muttered, "Yeah ... I'm beginning to wonder about that."

"What makes you wonder about that now?"

"I don't know ... and I'm not saying that I am an alcoholic ... but it seems like when all the shit comes down on me, it's always when I'm drinking. I don't know."

"So, what do you think? Do you think I have a problem? Am I an alcoholic?"

"Well," I said, choosing my words carefully, "it's a complicated issue, and I'm not sure I can say one way or another right now. I need to talk to you more about it and some other things before I say that. It looks like, from what you've told me, it's a possibility, but I'm not sure yet."

Jeremiah nodded.

I always believe chemically addicted people know they have problems, long before they admit it to others. The denial so often witnessed with these clients protects them from admitting problems to others, not necessarily from admitting problems to themselves.

If clients do not admit problems publicly, they do not have to take responsibility for their publicly admitted problems. Hence, I believed that Jeremiah knew he had problems with alcohol use; he simply could not admit it to me, a stranger who may have to report to the court someday or expect him to become accountable for finding remedy for the problems he admitted.

"How about next week we discuss this more, and maybe, if you're ready, discuss the war some."

"All right. War will be tough, though."

"I know. I've talked to others about it. That's some difficult stuff to talk about."

QUESTIONS

In this session, Jeremiah revealed much about his drinking history and how drinking affects his life, both in the present and over time. While it is still too early to make a final diagnosis, it is time to consider Jeremiah's condition. Therefore, find a *DSM-5* (APA, 2015) and locate the section on substance use disorder.

1. Beginning with the criteria for substance abuse, compare Jeremiah's information to those criteria. Does he meet the diagnostic criteria for substance abuse?
2. Then, compare his information to the criteria for substance dependence. Does he meet those criteria as well? Based on this initial finding, make your initial diagnosis of his drinking.
3. What about the mental health symptoms he described during the first two sessions? Do you believe Jeremiah qualifies for co-occurring disorders? If so, what is that second diagnosis?
4. At the end of the session, Jeremiah asked the author if he believed he was an alcoholic. The author did not answer him directly. What is your position on how the author handled that exchange? If you were in that

place, how would you have handled that question? Defend your position with information from the practice literature, your practice experience, and through discussion with student-colleagues.

Based on the information in this session, draw Jeremiah's three-generation genogram. What additional information do you need to complete the genogram?

5. Prochaska and DiClemente (1992) and DiClemente and Prochaska (1998) elaborated the Stages of Change model that posits five stages of change, called, from the earliest to the latest: precontemplation, contemplation, preparation/determination, action, and maintenance. I use these stages as assessment indicators of a client's level of motivation, for each diagnosed problem (Johnson, 2004). Based on outside readings about the stages of change/motivation:
   - At the conclusion of the first session, what stage do you believe Jeremiah was in for each diagnosis? Defend your decision.
   - At the end of the second session, what stage was Jeremiah in for each diagnosis? Defend your decision.
   - If you decide that a change of stage occurred between sessions one and two, what were the reasons for this change?
   - What would your plan be for the next session? Why?

SESSION THREE: TURNING POINT

[handwritten: Prep/Det. PTSD??]

Jeremiah returned for his third session the following week. However, on this day he was different. He had been drinking. He told me he drank before the first two sessions, too, but today I could tell. He appeared somewhat intoxicated. For the first time, I could smell alcohol on his breath, and his affect and mood were elevated. He was more excitable, awake, and talkative than before. Clearly, Jeremiah was more "social" when intoxicated. Perhaps this was the "Jeremiah" his family and close friends knew, instead of the serious, soft-spoken and guarded person I knew.

Why today, I wondered? Why did Jeremiah drink more before today's session and not earlier? Was he nervous about what I wanted to discuss? What I did know for sure was this session would be interesting.

There has always been widespread disagreement on whether to see an intoxicated client in therapy (Johnson, 2004). Many believe practitioners should not see intoxicated clients in therapy. These practitioners routinely terminate sessions with "substance abuse clients" if they admit to having a drink that day. Yet, often these same practitioners will meet with clients with non-substance abuse related problems after a three-martini business lunch. This practice is disingenuous at best and hypocritical at worst. From my perspective, intoxication is intoxication, whether people admit to having a substance use problem or not.

I do not automatically cancel an appointment with an intoxicated client. I make the decision based on three factors. First, can they participate in the session, or are they too intoxicated? Second, are client behaviors or attitudes so erratic practitioners may be at risk for an attack or some form of abuse during the session? Third, do the intoxicated clients need immediate medical attention?

If the answers to these questions indicate clients can understand and participate, are not erratic or dangerous, and not in medical crisis, then I proceed, even if for a few minutes. It can be enlightening to interview clients when they are intoxicated to compare their intoxicated and sober presentations. The differences can be astounding.

Therefore, I say go ahead and meet with intoxicated clients, but make sure to ask about their level of intoxication directly. Do not act as if you do not know; this makes you appear untrustworthy and naive in your client's eyes.

If you choose to cancel the appointment (as I have on occasion) or send them home early, do not just pack them off, especially if they drove to your office. If your intoxicated client has an accident after leaving your office, you could be liable. Instead, offer to call a taxi (even if your agency must pay), offer bus fare, or call someone to pick them up.

Moreover, if they are intoxicated and you choose to send them home, resist the urge to scold them as if they are misbehaving children. This is not the time for a lecture on why they should act more appropriately, why they are probably not suited for treatment, and how you will have to report this to their probation or parole officer.

If you feel compelled to lecture or scold—and you should never do it—wait until you see them again and they are sober. Simply cancel the appointment; make sure to write the next appointment time down in case their memory fails from blackout; and move on to your next session. If clients push you for an explanation, simply say that you can discuss it next session. Never try to reason with an intoxicated person.

Dealing with Jeremiah's Intoxication

Following my own advice, I asked Jeremiah about his drinking in my best, non-offended voice.

"Hey, Jeremiah, it looks to me like you've been drinking today. Is that right?"

"Yeah ... yeah, I did, but I'm not very drunk. I only had a few."

He was not agitated or threatening. He appeared to be coherent and ready for the session, so I proceeded. "Why did you drink today?"

"This stuff is hard, man. This is some serious shit we're talking about. ..."

"What shit?"

"Iraq ... the war, man."

He began crying, in the restrained way that men often do—a cross between the need for release and fear of humiliation. He was, after all, in his mind a tough combat veteran. Apparently, he pondered my suggestion last week about the planned content of this session. If you remember, I suggested we talk about his experience in combat and his drinking. He was showing me that his drinking was perhaps a way to gather the courage to discuss very serious and personal issues in his life and to deal with the stress and anxiety thinking and talking about it created. The two issues, drinking and combat, were fundamentally linked in Jeremiah's world.

"What about Iraq makes it so difficult to talk about?"

"What I saw ... what we had to do."

Jeremiah grew agitated, his eyes reddening from the salty sting of choked-back tears. He proceeded to tell me a frightening, ironic, and hauntingly tragic tale; one that could shake even the most hardened and seasoned therapist. I had heard horrible accounts of combat in wars from World War II to the Middle East from other clients and friends. I worked with Holocaust survivors and their children as a family therapist, but this story and its connection to Jeremiah's current dilemma was difficult to believe. He must have been imagining it, or was he?

Jeremiah recalled that his first tours of duty had been relatively uneventful. He spent a lot of time doing maintenance. Aside from the occasional attacks and other minor skirmishes, he was sheltered from most combat. When the third deployment came around, he figured it would be as uneventful as the others. Besides, he did not want to go home and face the fallout with the family over his joining the army in the first place. Jeremiah figured that one more year fixing vehicles would not be that bad. Before long, things changed.

Between his last tours while on dwell time at home, Jeremiah volunteered for combat for his next tour. The mission haunting him now turned out to be a door-to-door search-and-capture operation in a major Iraqi city. He soon found himself with colleagues in this city looking for enemy combatants, house to house.

At some point, they came under attack from Iraqi fighters: IED explosives, automatic gunfire, and grenade launchers. Jeremiah and mates ran for and found cover around a row of houses on a side street. As they proceeded down the street hoping to reenter the fray from a different angle, they came under small arms fire from neighboring homes.

"At that point, I lost my head ... and charged the first house I thought was shooting at us and shot open the door. We filled that house with hundreds of rounds as fast as we could, firing crazy. ... I was so scared."

After a few moments, the house went quiet. Jeremiah burst through the door, ready for more fighting, when the unthinkable became real.

"The only people in THAT HOUSE ... the house we cut to pieces ... was a young Iraqi mother and her children ... DEAD. I killed an innocent family ..." Jeremiah shouted, in between uncontrollable sobs and waves of nervous, shaking energy.

He looked to be in physical pain. He embodied agony, while having the kind of anguished emotional release one must have carrying and trying to hide hideous events that wounded him at his deepest level. Imagine, finally talking about something like this after more than 15 years of trying every means, including nearly killing himself with alcohol and other drugs and nearly killing his wife, to keep and survive with his secrets.

I sat silently and let him cry. Eventually he settled. He sat back in his chair and closed his eyes, as if seeing this woman, an Iraqi woman with long dark hair and two babies, lying dead in their own home; dead at Jeremiah's hands.

The connection between then and now, between the war and his family, between the Iraqi woman and her children in his memory and his Iraqi wife and twin daughters of his present, struck me hard. "Oh, my goodness," I thought, trying not to change facial expression or body language, "this woman is his wife, and the kids are his kids, at least in his mind's eye."

After a few moments, Jeremiah sat up and continued.

"We made a decision, but it wasn't that deliberate, you know. It's not as if we had a big discussion and took a vote. It was faster than that ... you don't have time to decide in a firefight. Shit, man, we were being fired on from all angles, and somebody pointed at that house and we took it apart. And there was this woman ... where I wish she hadn't been."

He paused and took a deep breath, almost as if he was sucking up the courage to go on with the story. He looked me straight in the eye: "I cut them down ... just cut them down. ..."

He stopped crying. He suddenly seemed clearer, as if he simply walled off his emotions from the specifics of the story. Telling the story as he remembered it, his emotions were intense, agonizing, and deep, but when he talked about the story, there was no obvious sorrow, no emotion, just calm, matter-of-fact words. He looked as if he were back in the war, with the focused and unemotional look of a combat veteran. To recover in the moment, Jeremiah seemed to have cut himself off from his feelings about being a player in the event. Perhaps this is how it had to be for Jeremiah to live. Maybe this was a "normal" adaptive reaction to living through the horrors of the war.

I could not know for sure. I had not been there, or in any combat situation. It would have been easy for me to judge him. I could not allow that to happen at this vulnerable moment in Jeremiah's life. At that moment, I was the only person alive he had ever told about this incident.

I cannot say with certainty this event happened the way Jeremiah described. My guess is that it did. Something, or a series of horrific things, happened.

Whatever happened on that day in the streets of Iraq was not the issue. The issue for Jeremiah was what he remembered and believed happened. His world revolved around his memory of a very specific, traumatic event that found him killing an Iraqi woman and her children during the war. His perception of that event and its obvious connection to his present life, emotional state, and more importantly, to shooting at another Iraqi woman (Fiona) who also happens to have his two children, was his lived reality. Historical accuracy always takes a backseat to memory and perception of events. This became a focus of our future work together.

Jeremiah's Major Conflict
"Jeremiah, as you tell me this story today, how do you feel?"

"Oh, man, ... when I think about it, it's bad. I don't know how to feel about it. I did what I had to do, but look what I did ... It was them or us ... what could I do? I killed them, but didn't know it was them I was killing. I was scared and somebody from that house ... I thought ... was trying to kill us. You'd have done the same thing, right?"

"I can't say what I would have done, since I've never been in that spot. You thought it was whoever was in that house or you. It was war ... did you have any other choice?"

"NO," he shouted, "I had no choice. The choice I made was to volunteer for combat ... that damned mission. I couldn't let whoever was shooting kill me or anybody else."

In this moment, Jeremiah had revealed the identity of his "traveling partners." He suffered from a divide between duty and ethics, what most soldiers in battle must face. On the one hand, he killed a woman and her children; on the other hand, he was a soldier in war, trained and paid to kill the enemy.

While he understood his duty, he suffered all these years with the guilt and shame associated with performing his duty. It haunted him for more than 15 years. He has worked full time and lived since that day, trying to bottle his experiences and feelings deep inside, hoping they would go away. They did not. Perhaps keeping his secrets was destroying him.

He spent our remaining time talking about his overwhelming guilt, the intense feelings he experienced since that day in Iraq, and how he discovered that alcohol and painkillers muted the intensity of his feelings and temporarily eased his internal conflict.

We discussed the devastating impact this had on his life and how he felt he could never tell anyone—not family, friends, or fellow veterans. He felt alone with his memories, guilt, shame, and nightmares; alcohol, painkillers, and the open road. Then, he identified perhaps the major source of his turmoil.

"How do I ever tell my wife what I did to an innocent woman and her children ... her people, for God's sake?"

"How could I ever tell her that I did that?"

As the session ended, I was concerned about Jeremiah's safety. He no longer appeared intoxicated. I suppose 90 minutes of this level of intensity took care of that. I had other worries. Given the intensity of the story and his feelings, his drinking, and access to weapons, I wondered about his suicide potential.

By the end of the session, he seemed calm, almost peaceful. He did not appear to be a candidate for suicide. Perhaps finally telling his story began the process of lifting his burden. Yet, my professional responsibility was to ensure, to the best of my ability, that Jeremiah was not about to kill himself.

When it comes to suicide risk, I ask about it directly and concretely. In this case, I believed he was a risk. He had access to weapons, drank and used drugs to intoxication, was male, had experienced significant trauma, had pending serious legal issues, and most importantly, lived a socially isolated life, with no friends, an estranged wife, and distant, tense, and cut-off family relationships. Beyond me, he had no source of support or resilience to fall back on.

My concerns were mitigated some because he had no apparent history of suicide attempts and he seemed dedicated and committed to his wife and family. I needed to screen him for suicide risk that day and in the future. He was treading through an emotional and experiential minefield. This combination of life circumstances could be lethal if not attended to regularly.

"Jeremiah, I have to ask. Given your circumstances and all, are you thinking about killing or harming yourself?"

"No, man. I have a family and kids. I'd never do that to them."

"Have you ever thought about it?"

"No ... I told you that before. I love my family. After living through the war and all, I want to live. Hell, I just want things to be normal. So no, don't worry. I'll be all right."

"Okay. If anything changes, you can call here, or the people at this number (local hotline) if you can't reach me."

He nodded.

As someone who regularly treats people with alcohol problems, I had a portable breathalyzer in my office. He agreed to have his blood alcohol level (BAL) tested before leaving to ensure that he was able to legally drive home. His BAL fell below the legal limit of the era, so he was safe to drive himself.

Jeremiah shook my hand, heaved a big sigh, wiped his eyes, and left. Since one can never be sure about suicide risk, I hoped to see him again.

CASE SUMMARY

In this case, I describe Jeremiah and his current situation in significant detail. This account of my work with Jeremiah takes you through the first three sessions of what became a 13-month professional relationship. While Jeremiah's case was unique because of his unusual and dramatic war experiences, how our relationship developed was not. That is, by focusing on rapport and engagement during the early stages of therapy instead of confrontation, intervention planning, and change, even mandated and/or coerced clients can progress from what some would call resistant to what I call engaged, willing partners in the therapeutic process.

From the point where Jeremiah and I began, to the end of the third session, he had changed. No, he had not stopped drinking or resolved his issues, but he had changed. His change began when he shared his story. He was no longer in the predicament of being alone with his demons and feeling hopeless that his life will never be different. He was developing hope. He had demonstrated, by his willingness to return each week and delve into intimate personal experiences and feelings, that he had hope for his future, that his life could be different in the future. He was becoming "hooked" on possibility, instead of overwhelmed by problems and limitations. He was beginning to realize that he could be an agent for positive change in his life. The empowerment process had begun.

However, our work is not complete—not even close. This is where you come in. It is now your task to work with Jeremiah and his demons. As you move forward planning the remainder of the case, do not be fooled into believing that the level of engagement and commitment Jeremiah exhibited to this point is permanent. It is one thing to engage clients to the point where they will relive and relate their lives. This is the easy part. It is a different task to get Jeremiah to deepen his commitment to himself and his family and take concrete steps toward a new life.

Under your care, Jeremiah is about to confront his own dilemma of change (Johnson, 2004). That is, he has choices, none of which appear promising from his perspective at this moment in his life. It is your job as practitioners to help him find his way from this point forward, keeping in mind that the relationship will have to build with every step of the process, or treatment will likely fail.

This is the point in Jeremiah's case where you take over. What happens next? I pass Jeremiah to you for completion. Good luck!

ASSESSMENT, DIAGNOSES, AND TREATMENT PLANNING

QUESTIONS

1. Finish drawing the three-generation genogram that you began earlier. Also, develop an eco-map that best represents Jeremiah's involvement with multiple social systems and organizations in his environment.
2. Make a list, with supporting evidence, of the main issues in Jeremiah's life at this moment. Include in that enumeration a list of his personal and environmental strengths that pertain to each of the issues you listed.

3. Next, develop and write a comprehensive narrative assessment of Jeremiah's life, family, social support, culture, and his environment. Your narrative assessment should reflect the multisystemic information gleaned from him during his three sessions. The multisystemic narrative assessment becomes the client's case history report (Johnson, 2004) and includes a comprehensive diagnostic statement that integrates essential client information into a coherent description of their life, history, and current circumstances. The case history report concludes with a *DSM* diagnosis (or, in this case, perhaps multiple diagnoses).

The case history report should lead directly to a written initial treatment plan (Johnson, 2004) that is understandable and agreeable to your client. This plan should include your client as a full partner in the process. This will be especially important in Jeremiah's case, given the importance of African American males being partners in the treatment process. There are many formats available to develop treatment plans (Johnson, 2004) use whatever format you want to enhance your learning in this case.

INTERVENTION PLANNING AND IMPLEMENTATION

Based on the comprehensive case history report and written treatment plan developed above, it is now time to decide on intervention strategies. List each intervention you would use in your work with Jeremiah. Specifically, for each intervention, include the target issue, intervention, and modality (i.e., group therapy) you chose and the theoretical justification for each.

1. What other options might be available should these interventions prove ineffective?
2. What does the latest empirical evidence in the field suggest for each target issue? How does this evidence match with your intervention strategies?
3. When developing treatment approaches, do not overlook nontraditional approaches and approaches that target multiple systemic levels (i.e., individual, family, community, advocacy, etc.).
4. What factors and strategies will you use to build trust and engagement during the intervention phases of your work? How will you assist Jeremiah as his motivation for change waxes and wanes over the coming weeks and months?

TERMINATION, AFTERCARE, AND FOLLOW-UP

Preparing for termination begins early in the treatment process. Proper termination includes many factors, besides how your client progresses in treatment. Hence, this exercise will help you think about the various issues that go into successful termination, aftercare, and follow-up.

1. List and explain the general factors to consider in developing a successful aftercare plan for substance abusing clients.
2. List and explain the issues in Jeremiah's life to consider when planning for termination and aftercare.
3. What indicators (Jeremiah's progress in treatment) will you use to determine when it is an appropriate time for termination?
4. Plan a specific strategy for termination, aftercare, and follow-up that best fits Jeremiah's reality and professional standards of practice. What does the latest empirical evidence in the field say about these issues?

REFERENCES

American Psychiatric Association. (2015). *Diagnostic and statistical manual of mental disorders* (5th ed.). Author.

Bowen, M. (1985). *Family therapy in clinical practice*. Aronson.

Connors, G. J., Donovan, D. M., & DiClemente, C. C. (2001). *Selecting and planning interventions: Substance abuse treatment and the stages of change*. Guilford Press.

DiClemente, C. C., & Prochaska, J. O. (1998). Toward a comprehensive, transtheoretical model of change: Stages of change and addictive behaviors. In W. R. Miller & N. Heather (Eds.), *Treating addictive behaviors* (2nd ed., pp. 3–24). Plenum Press.

Johnson, J. L. (2004). *Fundamentals of substance abuse practice*. Thomson-Brooks/Cole.

Miller, W. R., & Rollnick, S. (2002). *Motivational interviewing: Preparing people to change addictive behavior* (2nd ed.). Guilford Press.

Prochaska, J. O., & DiClemente, C. C. (1992). Stages of change in the modification of problem behaviors. In M. Hersen, R. M. Eisler, & P. M. Miller (Eds.), *Progress in behavior modification* (Vol. 28, pp. 183–218). Sycamore.

Richardlin, A. J. (1992). Therapy with African American men. *Families in Society: The Journal of Contemporary Human Services*, 350–355.

Rooney, R. H. (2002). Working with involuntary clients. In A. R. Roberts & G. J. Greene (Eds.), *Social workers' desk reference* (pp. 709–716). Oxford University Press.

Rooney, R. H. (1992). *Strategies for working with involuntary clients*. Columbia University Press.

CHAPTER 3

Juan or John
A Case of Lost Racial Identity

Salvador Lopez-Arias

ALLOW ME TO introduce you to Juan, a 42-year-old Mexican American male with multiple problems and issues in his life. It is easy to assume the friendly looking male waiting patiently in the waiting room will be like so many others I have treated over my nearly 30-year career. Based on the information on his intake sheet, Juan seemed like so many others. I was wrong. First off, Juan wanted to be called John. Secondly, he became the first Latino client who preferred a white male therapist instead of myself, a well-experienced Mexican American social worker. Juan's case becomes even more interesting and challenging after that inauspicious beginning.

As you progress through Juan's life challenges, I have included a series of questions designed to guide and challenge your thinking. For the best learning experience, please stop and work through the questions as they arise.

INTRODUCTION

In my nearly 30 years as a therapist specializing in treating substance use and mental health disorders, I have encountered clients from diverse backgrounds and attitudes and with multiple problems in their lives. After seeing hundreds, if not thousands, of clients, it would be easy for me to believe I've seen it all. Working in this profession with people having different presentation and problems, struggling to find a better, more effective way of living in their world, is one of the reasons I love the helping profession. I find each case different and unique, even if they appear similar on their face. This case proved to me that I have, in fact, not seen it all.

The challenge for practitioners is to avoid letting our experience gained over the years lull us into believing clients are the same; to avoid the tendency to stereotype clients by problem type, racial, or ethnic backgrounds, or any other factor. In other words, therapy cannot be approached from a "one-size-fits-all" approach. The challenge is to see each client as unique, to note similarities across clients but constantly and curiously search every client's background and history looking for exceptions, differences, and unique combinations of problems, strengths, and opportunities different from all other "similar" appearing clients.

Juan, a Latino male who demanded I call him John, is no exception. From the beginning, John presented many issues and attitudes consistent across people struggling with substance use disorders and a lifetime of racial and ethnic mistreatment and exclusion. It would have been easy to approach him in that way. To have done so would have been arrogant, born of a negative practice privilege developed through years of experience. This approach comes from a place of privilege that says I have all the answers for John—despite not knowing him—if only he would listen.

Practitioners should treat each client's worldview, or cultural practices, as unique. Since everyone's worldview is developed in specific and individualized social environments, each person's perspectives are unique. A practitioner comfortable in multicultural settings with diverse clients must be aware of such differences and the impact these differences have on people's life experience and clinical presentation. We then must develop the interpersonal and clinical skills necessary to discover these unique features. These factors (and more) affect a client's willingness to engage in therapy and their readiness to change.

The need for individualization, while true for every client, is especially true with clients from US minority backgrounds. Hence, it is crucial to conceptualize minority clients from a holistic perspective while assessing how their life interacts with oppressive events (e.g., sexism, racism, and heterosexism, homophobia) and the extent to which these issues should be addressed in therapy. Approaching minority clients in this way can lead to a stronger working alliance, often offering a better chance for change.

Moreover, the professional literature states clinical practice with substance use–disordered clients can be more difficult than practice in other specific areas (DiClemente, Nidecker, & Bellack, 2008). However, DiClemente and Velasquez (2002) contend these difficulties diminish if practitioners employ a readiness, or stages-of-change, approach. According to the authors, a stage-of-change approach helps hesitant, ambivalent, and apparently resistant clients become aware of the possibility of and the need to change (DiClemente & Velasquez, 2002).

MEETING JUAN (OR JOHN)

It was late on Friday afternoon. After a long week, I was about to head home for a weekend with my family. As I was clearing my desk of paperwork, I received a call from our front desk. The receptionist asked if I would be willing to see one more client before I left for the weekend. My colleague was supposed to see this client, but he needed to leave to attend to a family emergency at the local hospital.

When I readily agreed to stay and help, our staff member told me about an apparent problem. It appears this client was "hesitant" to see a Latino therapist. I am a native of Mexico, having lived in the United States for nearly 30 years. This qualifies me as a "Latino" therapist. Anticipating problems with what I thought was going to be a white, male client, I offered to perform the initial intake session and transfer the case back to my colleague, a white male therapist. On multiple occasions, majority clients expressed hesitancy at the prospect of seeing a minority clinician. I figured this would be a case of "more of the same."

When I entered the waiting area, to my surprise, sitting alone in the room was a man I perceived to be of Latin descent waiting for his intake session. This was odd. Maybe my new client was in the bathroom and this gentleman was waiting for somebody else. Or perhaps my visual perception of this man's ethnicity was wrong.

When it was clear nobody else was waiting, I warmly greeted the gentleman and escorted him to my office, wondering about the hesitancy mentioned by our receptionist. Perhaps she misunderstood him. Maybe he was hesitant to see a white therapist! That would have been more typical.

On his admission form, my new client wrote his name—Juan. When I addressed him as "Juan," he sternly said he preferred to be called "John." Further, he said he intended to legally change his name to John because he was "tired" of people calling him Juan.

I realized I'd made a mistake. Despite him stating his name was Juan on the form, I failed to ask him what he preferred to be called. Everyone likes to be called by the name or nickname they prefer. I assumed what he wrote was his preference. I took away his freedom to be called what he wants when I addressed him directly as Juan without asking. Experienced practitioners, like I claim to be, understand the importance—even the power—of a positive first impression in successful client engagement (Johnson, 2004). I might have created another hurdle to overcome.

After shaking hands and entering my small, yet comfortable, office, John immediately claimed he did not need therapy for drinking, and he especially did not need to see me—for anything.

"I'm not one of those Mexicans that can't speak English."

I reassured John that although I was Mexican American and bilingual, most of my clients were white and I could work with him if he wanted. John seemed surprised. I guess he never imagined that whites would be comfortable working with a Mexican American therapist. After asking for my credentials and experience, he agreed to proceed.

QUESTIONS

1. Given what you know about John/Juan, what issues would you consider as you prepared to meet him for the first time?
2. How would you prepare yourself to overcome the issues described to this point?
3. Before reading the next section, how do you approach apparently hostile or resistant clients in your practice?

I began by asking about the circumstances of his referral to our center. Instead of answering, he quickly interrupted to ask more about my qualifications and experience. Refusing to look up, John stared, almost unconvinced, that I, a Mexican American male, could possibly have the qualifications and experience to be a real professional therapist. He did everything except accuse me of faking my credentials.

Now, I have experienced this many time before, but usually from white clients. Never had I felt such distrust, disrespect, and uncertainty from a Latino client. Typically, Latino clients are overjoyed—at least pleased—to see my brown skin and hear my familiar accent. Apparently, John was going to be an unusual challenge.

It is not uncommon for clients to challenge their new therapist, especially if they are from a different racial, ethnic, and/or gender background than the practitioner. This is often a by-product of years of ill treatment by the majority, the result of personal negative implicit bias or actual negative life experiences. I always expect some level of mistrust from any new client. After all, as a new person in their life, my job is to be "nosy" by asking probing questions about their personal lives, problems, and circumstances. The difference here was John's intense mistrust in me because I am a Latino male. As I stated earlier, this seemed unusual coming from a minority client toward a minority therapist from a similar ethnic group.

What's in a Name? John or Juan?

I immediately wanted to learn about how John came to distance himself, even despise, his ethnic heritage. As a proud Mexican American person, his hard work to disavow his Mexican heritage, especially in front of me, was unsettling. He went so far as to change his name from Juan to John in an apparent effort to either be white, or American, or both.

In his important work, Cross (1978) discusses four stages of African American (and other minority) racial development. Included among these developmental identity formation stages are the pre-encounter, encounter, immersion/emersion, internalization, and commitment stages. According to Cross (1978), people often begin in the pre-encounter stage (denial of heritage, disparaging ethnic or racial background, anger, hostility, etc.) and hopefully proceed to the final stage of commitment, or pride and connection to one's heritage, background, and people. In the final stage, clients of color develop a more secure sense of self as an individual and group member while developing an individual plan of action or a sense of commitment to the well-being of their group (Cross, 1978).

According to Bridges (2011), as people move through these stages, their identity develops from non-ethnocentric to ethnocentric. The high level of negative exposure and stereotypical representations of minorities in the environment and the media often lead people to identify with the majority. However, as they are unable to belong to the majority, they begin identifying with their own group. This is especially true as people are exposed to positive messages or role modeling from members of their own cultural or ethnic group, leading to a more ethnocentric identity.

Although Cross's model focused mostly on African American identity processes like Helms (1990), I believe it addresses identity development for members of most ethnic, racial, or otherwise oppressed groups in the United States, struggling to navigate a majority-centered society.

While processing John's intense reaction to me, I came to realize in many ways his worldview made good survival sense. Recently, the political rhetoric in the United States has portrayed Mexican Americans as hostile and problematic, an existential threat to white American life. Perhaps this was driving his anger.

Yet, John's hostility seemed different, coming from a deeper place. He did not fit the background of someone afraid of the atmosphere. He was older, male, and since he was born in the United States, was not undocumented. Besides, he did not present as angry at the United States or the hurtful rhetoric ... he seemed to agree with it!

Sensing this unique and different situation, I grew curious about what life experiences, lack of development, or other influences worked on this man over his lifetime to generate this level of hostility and discomfort with himself, expressed through his mistrust and hostility toward me.

Quickly, I was left deciding what to do and how to handle this issue. One thing for sure, I strongly believe in my responsibility to be a role model, especially in circumstances like this. I intended to role model for John what it means to be a healthy Mexican American male, made more difficult since he not only held negative views of Mexicans, Mexican Americans, and Latino males, but Latinos in general.

> **QUESTIONS**
>
> 1. Before moving ahead with the case, consider the issues pertaining to building client rapport and engagement. What is your approach to this issue, and to what importance do you give professional relationship building?
> 2. What are the most important factors in client engagement?
> 3. What percentage of your time do you spend working on and/or practicing your engagement skills? List several ways that you can improve or practice engagement skills.
> 4. Given your personal and professional heritage and background, how would you approach someone as conflicted as John? What strengths do you bring, and what would be the most significant barriers given John's presentation and your person?

APPROACHING JOHN IN THERAPY

Given all the apparent complexities of John's life, I considered how best to approach him. In other words, how can I approach his circumstances in a way that would give John the best chance for success?

Adding to his apparent difficulty with me, or perhaps because of it, over time John was regularly late for sessions. Many practitioners find this irritating, leading some to immediately label tardy clients as resistant to treatment. I believe being late can be a sign of resistance or a lack of engagement or trust. This was the case between John and me. For others, according to their cultural background, time is not as important and being late is acceptable. For clients lacking resources and transportation and having significant life difficulties, it can be difficult for these clients to get anywhere "on time." I try to be understanding and compassionate and do not mention lateness unless it becomes obvious it is a sign of resistance.

He exhibited other difficult signs early in our relationship. For example, he consistently challenged nearly everything I asked or said. He often referenced his "bad temper," claiming his wife and coworkers feared his volatile temper. Whenever I offered feedback, John became evasive and defensive, often responding with, "I knew that," or by disagreeing. He seemed to enjoy arguing with me about nearly everything. For much of our time together, John tried to negate my observations, even observations he requested.

Some clients exhibit anxiety, anger, or fear when they feel powerless as a way to gain power and control over their environment. This seemed to be the case with John. He appeared committed to doing whatever he could to maintain a sense of control over our conversation, even threatening a bad temper to keep me on guard.

As stated earlier, John's worldview seemed dominated by the perspective of the US majority. He had internalized many of the negative stereotypes and attitudes held by the majority about his people and background. According to Cross (1978), people with this level of hostility often express themselves by denigrating their own people, often trying to be "White" or to pass as white.

John presented as a Mexican American male trying his utmost to avoid being labeled as such. He clearly saw others as "immigrants" but seemed to have no understanding of his own heritage. As a result of his strictly conservative, almost bigoted, political position regarding immigrants and minorities, John sounded more like a stereotypical right-wing European American male than a Mexican American from an immigrant family who grew up poor in the Midwest.

John appeared to exemplify how some people's internalized shame leads to an effort to distance themselves from their background. I have often seen this with clients experiencing stigma from poverty, family and physical/sexual abuse, family or personal substance use and abuse, sexual orientation, and race/culture.

He did not want to see a Latino therapist because of his internalized belief that minorities were inferior. He desperately wanted to see himself as better, part of the majority American culture. He despised immigrants ("Why don't they go back to their own country?") especially those living in the United States illegally. He practiced ultraconservative politics and actively avoided Latinos in all aspects of his life.

John wanted to "fit in." He craved external approval and acceptance from White, middle-class Americans. His desires were so strong it made it impossible for him to associate with racial and/or ethnic groups deemed inferior by the majority. He sought distance from his Latino background to reduce the shame he felt because he was Latino. He felt as if he was an "outsider" in the United States, even though he was native born.

"Where do you feel like you fit in?" I asked.

"I used to feel good in church, but then they got so into helping the poor and minorities.... I'm tired of hearing about how they've suffered. Nobody ever helped me, and I made it just fine."

According to John, his social exclusion started early in life. In high school, John tried fitting in with the crowd, but was never accepted. He said he always felt "alone" in the small, Midwestern town where his grandmother lived and where he was raised.

Presently, John reported having few friends, with the exception a "couple of people" from church. In the past, he said his "so-called" friends had "taken advantage" of his friendship. This experience left a bad taste in his mouth. Hence, John did not want friends because he did not want those kinds of problems again.

"I don't know anyone worth trusting."

His disconnectedness and social isolation concerned me. People who have been bullied, mistreated in their families, or rejected and become socially isolated out of fear of anger often present grave risks for harm to self and others, through either suicide or homicide. Social isolation can lead to internal reinforcement of their trauma and possible destructive and violent behavior (Johnson, 2004).

So, is John a resistant client? Well, if you are the person being challenged, it certainly feels like it in the moment. I had to be careful to manage my reactions to his challenges and attitudes in a way that did not let him see or sense my rising sense of defensiveness. Regardless of years of experience, circumstances like these are difficult. Learning to manage oneself in the face of mistrust and suspicion is part of daily practice preparation and bettering oneself at handling our internal thoughts, feelings, and reactions without giving ourselves away is a career-long challenge (Johnson, 2004).

I expect a certain amount of ambivalence or resistance from new clients. Imagine sharing your most intimate life struggles with a stranger, someone who can alter your life (positively or negatively) based on what you tell them. For some, what we report to a referral source and/or the outcome of therapy may determine if they lose or keep a job, divorce or remain married, keep their freedom or be imprisoned, and/or retain custody of their children. It is unrealistic to expect or assume clients, especially when they are mandated to therapy, will enter a new therapeutic relationship ready to be honest and/or vulnerable.

All relationships take time to develop, especially therapeutic relationships. Trust with intimacy and vulnerability between therapist and client must be earned over time. It is important for clients to trust us and know we are trustworthy before investing in such a relationship. In fact, I believe it unhealthy for clients to become too vulnerable too soon before trust and safety develop. From a client's perspective, they generally have a lot to lose if they encounter anyone, especially professional helpers, who are untrustworthy.

Over the years, I have heard colleagues label clients as dishonest, worried about clients telling the "truth" about their lives. I think this is unfairly judgmental, especially early in the therapeutic relationship. My practice approach, based in the context described above, assumes clients will become more forthcoming when they are ready, when they develop the requisite level of trust in me, and sense that I have unconditional positive regard for them as people. When this begins to develop, clients almost naturally talk more truth about their lives and circumstances. Until that happens, clients will often tell us what they believe we want to hear instead of the truth.

These issues are often enhanced among people with substance use disorders. People with substance use disorders often suffer a level of shame, guilt, and stigma in their communities that inhibits how they approach life, including therapy (Carlson, 2006; Dunn, 2005; Room, Rehm, Trotter, Paglia, & Üstün, 2001). According to the World Health Organization (WHO), drug addiction was considered the most stigmatizing health condition, followed closely by alcohol addiction as the fourth most stigmatizing condition (Room, Rehm, Trotter, Paglia, & Üstün, 2001). This level of stigma and the resulting guilt and shame often leads clients to resist telling the truth about their behaviors and/or admitting to existing substance use problems. They are often left feeling vulnerable while avoiding the subject or becoming defensive.

I decided to approach John the same as I approach every client, regardless of the circumstances of their referral, or who they are or how they feel about themselves, their heritage, or in this case, my heritage, too. I work to develop a relationship while seeking to understand the context of their life, history, issues, and strengths as part of the process of establishing a therapeutic relationship based on mutual trust and agreeable goals (Johnson, 2004). Early on, I typically avoid confrontation or overt challenges. I simply ask questions, listen, and try to understand my client's lived experience.

Given John's personality, it would have been easy and professionally lazy to become frustrated. His behavior, beliefs, attitudes, and values were determined by his unique reaction to his life experience. I literally had nothing to do with who he had become. In other words, his mistrust of me had nothing to do with me. It was not personal. Understanding this truth allows me to work with hostile clients. Their attitudes and behaviors are what life has taught them. It's about survival, not about us.

Instead of labeling John as resistant, I decided to view him as vulnerable, sensing his feelings that his life and future were out of his control. As I stated earlier, John must have good, real reasons to feel how he does. It is my job to get him to share them with me.

QUESTION

As we proceed through the remainder of the case, draw John's three-generation genogram based on the forthcoming information gathered over the following sessions.

Our Work Begins: John and Lisa's Marriage

Over the course of our first meeting, John's suspicion about me seemed to lessen. As I sensed his change of attitude, I began slowly and patiently inquiring about his life.

John (or Juan) presented as a 42-year-old Latino male from a Christian, Catholic background. He had been married to his wife, Lisa, for nearly 24 years. The couple recently separated after an intense argument turned physical. From the beginning, John insisted he had no problems with alcohol or drugs, only his marriage. To honor his desire to begin with his marriage, I moved to open the conversation and see how far he would take it.

"You know, my marriage is my biggest problem … has been for years. If it wasn't for that, I probably wouldn't drink at all."

I find it interesting—and perhaps telling—that John mentioned his "drinking" several times early in our first session, especially since I never asked him about it. Hopefully, joining with him around his marriage would help him decide to return, when I would have plenty of time to ask about his drinking.

"What do you want to do about your marriage?" I asked.

"I would like help figuring out how to make it better, make it work like it used to. I really want to stay with Lisa, but I don't want any more physical stuff going on."

Physical? Not only did he bring up his drinking without prompting, but now he mentioned problems in his marriage related to "getting physical." These unprompted revelations suggested either he was settling in therapy with me, or he was feeling so much internal pressure he could not hold it in any longer.

"How often do you two get physical?"

After a long hesitation, John replied, "Oh … probably every other week or so. Most of the time I'm defending myself. She gets so pissed off and explodes at me … hitting, kicking, punching. …"

"And when was the last time?"

"Monday night" (two days prior to this meeting)," he said, looking down and away in apparent embarrassment.

Domestic Violence

Now that John had settled into our conversation, I believed it time to approach his earlier mention of possible domestic violence between Lisa and himself. John seemed willing to talk freely about his marital troubles, so I delved more deeply into them.

John said his frustration "with everything … Lisa, my job … you name it" led to daily, loud, and hostile arguments with Lisa. Lately, the situation went from bad to worse.

"What do you mean, John? What went from bad to worse?"

"The whole thing … our marriage … seems to be coming to a head. Everything I do now leads to a fight," he said.

"Like what?"

"She doesn't even want me to have a drink anymore. I'm nicer to her, more patient when I have a few drinks. She never used to care if I drank, but lately that's changed. Heck, she even used to have drinks after work with me but now, I guess she's changed her mind."

After refusing to discuss his drinking earlier, I was surprised he brought it up again. This will give me an opening to collect a more thorough history when the time is right. Now, I wanted to see how far he would go discussing his drinking.

Given that he brought up the subject and my questions would be in the context of discussing his marriage, I felt good about my chances of learning more now.

"When did Lisa change her mind about your having a few drinks?"

"Oh, that just happened ... recently. I don't get her sometimes. Can't please her no matter what I do ..."

"Did something happen that caused her to change her mind?"

"I don't know ... couple times lately I was short tempered, impatient. She probably blamed it on alcohol. But it's not a problem ... not a problem ..."

John said he normally drank only "two to three times a week." When he drank, John claimed he would only have "one or two beers" as a way to relax after a long day of work or when Lisa "got under my skin." He said he rarely drank to intoxication and reiterated his belief that his drinking was not a problem, but a needed relief from all the stresses in life.

I decided to leave drinking and return to the conversation about his marriage. I was beginning to feel confident John would return for further sessions, based on his willingness, so far, to discuss highly personal issues. I decided to gamble on my belief that we would have more time to dive further into his drinking history later.

"Okay, John, you were talking about your marriage and the problems you have with Lisa. How does your trying to help her turn nasty from time to time?"

"Hell, I don't know. I can't figure the woman out. She is really unpredictable ... good one minute and mean the next."

According to John, nearly anything, including his efforts to help her, started an argument which would sometimes lead to a physical fight. "Out of the blue," Lisa would start slapping and hitting him while he was helping her to stand up or lie down. She would angrily refuse food and drink, even throwing it on the floor to show her disgust at his cooking prowess. John claimed she would "throw things" at him when her pain worsened if he was either too slow to help or complaining about having to help. This often led to the couple yelling at each other, sometimes "nose to nose."

"What do you do when she hits you?"

John appeared to think deeply about my question or his answer. I was not sure if talking about this bothered him, or he was shaping his answer to make him look like the victim, or if he was in fact the victim.

"Occasionally, very occasionally ... I have to defend myself."

"What do you mean, defend yourself?"

"Sometimes I just can't take it. I try to be a nice guy ... I mean, she's in a lot of pain. But I just can't take her hitting me."

Although he was "nicer" to her when he drank, according to John, often their arguments would escalate if she hit him. He could also trigger a physical altercation if he refused to apologize for doing something wrong, even if he did not know what he did that was wrong. Her hitting and he physically defending himself gradually became the norm over time.

"How long has this been going on?"

"Oh ... for years. I'll bet we've been doing this for five or six years."

"To clarify: when you say 'defend yourself,' what does that mean specifically?"

John defined "defending himself" as usually grabbing her with the necessary force to stop from being slapped and hit in the face. He claimed he "never" hit her back but stopped her from hitting him.

"When is the last time it got physical?"

"Two days ago," he said. "It was a bad one, too."

According to John, Lisa became angry "over something ... I don't know what," and began slapping him about the face and neck. Apparently, during this event, John "grabbed" her with such force, he "accidentally" dislocated her shoulder.

"What did you do after that?" I asked, assuming he took her to the hospital or called someone for help.

"I left. I was still so angry with her that I was afraid what I would do if she said anything else."

He paused. That's why I came here. I don't know if I can be with her anymore, but I feel like I have to be with her."

"You left for the night, or moved out?"

"I sort of moved out ..."

Lisa wanted John to come home, but he refuses to move back home, although he visits to help her daily. John said this incident frightened him, bringing back memories of his father.

"I'm afraid I might let her turn me into my father," he said.

While John said he "wanted" to return home to Lisa, he said the couple would "probably" need therapy before that could happen. Without help, John believed they would certainly have another physical altercation, and he said he did not want that to happen again.

QUESTIONS

John just described an incidence of apparent domestic violence that recently occurred between his wife and himself.

1. Given this information, what next steps would you take, both immediately and over the remainder of the session?
2. What does the current professional literature have to say about this incidence arising early in therapy?
3. What does your profession's Code of Professional Ethics say about how to handle this circumstance in treatment?
4. What is your opinion about how the author proceeds?

Given the alarming revelations about domestic violence, it was important for me to understand the situation to determine its severity and whether outside protective intervention was required. To accomplish this, I thought it important to gather more information about his relationship with Lisa and its history to help me understand how their marriage reached this point of crisis.

It appears John was born and raised in the southwest United States. At age 12, he moved with his paternal grandmother to the Midwest, where he continues to live. After dropping out of high school and receiving his GED, John met Lisa while both attended a local community college. They married when John was 18 and Lisa 19, after Lisa became pregnant. Unfortunately, she miscarried shortly after their marriage. They have no other children.

John said he always had "problems" with Lisa's extended family, especially his in-laws. He was Mexican American, and his wife was white. According to John, Lisa's family did not approve of her marrying a Mexican. John believed most of his marital problems resulted from misunderstandings between Lisa and himself and her family's constant efforts to separate them.

John admitted feeling "distant" from his wife but insisted he did not want a divorce. While the couple argued a lot and, according to John, both became physically abusive, he "definitely" wanted his marriage to survive. Neither John nor Lisa believes in divorce on religious grounds.

"We're gonna have to find a way to make this work," John sighed.

I wondered if the marriage had always been difficult, or if something happened or changed over the years.

According to John, the first years of marriage were "good." He reported no "big" problems between them, they had "a lot" of fun, and seemed to enjoy each other's company. Their troubles began 12 years earlier, right after Lisa was badly injured in a car accident, leaving her disabled with back and neck injuries. While her injuries do not limit her mobility, Lisa's recurrent and chronic pain, along with the effects of significant doses of pain medication, caused problems, John said.

"I just got tired of her sleeping all the time … seems like she was always either in a trance or angry, loud, and violent," he said. "She would stay in bed for days. Doctors told me there was no physical reason to be in bed all the time. Yes … she had pain, but she could move."

"How'd you handle it?" I asked

"It really pissed me off. I started really resenting her lying there, demanding I wait on her … then complaining when I did. I couldn't take it anymore."

John went on to talk about his coming to resent being "stuck" at home, taking care of her every need. "I'm so tired of being her nursemaid."

"What do you mean?"

"I mean, she says she's disabled, but she gets around fine when she wants too. She's always complaining about being depressed, but she uses so much medication I don't know how she couldn't be depressed, or at least asleep."

According to John, Lisa "always" says she is depressed. In addition, he claims she overuses pain medication, causing her to be lethargic and disinterested in anything besides being in bed and watching television. John resented being obligated to take care of her, especially since he claims she does little to take care of him, including and especially, sexually.

"Have you ever thought about leaving her?"

"Oh, yeah, I have … many times. There have been days and nights where I actually packed a bag ready to leave … and then …"

"Then what?"

John was convinced he was in a bind. On the one hand, he wanted to leave, even knew he should leave because their relationship was unhealthy. Yet, whenever he thought seriously about it, he began "feeling sorry for her." This dilemma was compounded because of his belief he would be rejected by his church if he divorced her. Hence, he always stayed.

"I'm not sure anymore if I love her … or feel sorry for her," he said.

I was unsure if he pitied her, or himself. I had so many questions for John. For example, what or who would constitute his support system if he decided to seek a divorce from Lisa? Does he have friends, family, colleagues on the job who could help him during what would be a difficult time? Perhaps he stayed not out of sympathy for her, but because she was all he had in life. These were all issues to discover in the future.

Religion

Since John mentioned how important his church was to him, I wondered if his faith affected how he approached marriage and/or how he handled his marital issues and problems. Many practitioners do not broach the subject of religion and faith with clients, outside of some form of religious or faith-based counseling. I am not talking here about helping someone find or enhance their faith, nor am I talking about imposing my personal religion or religious beliefs onto clients. I am talking about helping clients discuss and explore their religious or spiritual beliefs and practices and how these shape their personal worldview. A person's faith tradition is central to their personal worldview (Johnson & Grant, 2005). This is especially true with clients who report struggles specifically related to religion and faith, as John did early in our first session. Earlier he discussed problems and issues related to his church and its practices. This is an important issue because John seemed to rely on his church as a significant source of belonging and social support.

According to John, his Catholic faith and his church were important. He attended mass at least twice per week, as well as other activities. Many weeks, John reported Lisa and he attended some activity at church three to four times. In the past, John and Lisa found the church and its people to be sources of support and comfort. Lately, this changed. John said he was having problems with many of his church's positions and activities. Moreover, John claimed that his faith "wasn't working" for him like it used to. He used to find peace, but no longer.

"What do you mean?" I inquired.

"I used to believe God loved me … now, I know that can't be true."

Instead of finding solace and acceptance, John found pain in his religious life. I wondered where his belief system originated. Often, it begins with people's family of origin.

John's Family of Origin

At this time, I thought it better to ease the tension in the room and inquire about his family of origin and how it was for him growing up. Not only do clients find this easier to discuss, but it provides so many clues about how they think, feel, believe, and act that it becomes vital to successful therapy. Moreover, learning about a client's upbringing gives clues about how they manage marriage, religion, and other significant issues in their adult life. I find clients, even the most suspicious, will provide family information freely while providing a lot of relevant information to help in the assessment of many areas of their lives.

"If it's okay with you John, let's take a minute and talk about your family growing up."

Instead of relaxing, as I expected, he physically recoiled at my suggestion. "I hate talking about them …"

I guess this proves there are exceptions to every practice "rule."

Apparently, John had "lost touch" with his family many years earlier, by choice. He grew up the youngest of five children, and there was a 12-year age difference between him and his next oldest sibling. He claimed he barely knew his older siblings because of the age difference.

As a child, John said he was "close" to his sister (next eldest sibling) since she was his de facto parent. His relationship with his sister basically ended when she met and married the "first man that came along." John believed she did this because their father had been especially hard on her and she wanted to escape the family home.

By the time John turned 10 years old, he was living alone with his father, whom John called "an emotionally and physically abusive" man. John's father was a Korean War veteran who treated his children as if they were soldiers, demanding respect and compliance, and physically and verbally punishing any missteps or normal childhood behavior.

John's father reportedly physically abused his mother, who died of cancer when John was 10 years old. John's father was an impatient and short-tempered man who also physically abused him. Moreover, he developed a "bad" alcohol problem over the years. His father's heavy and constant drinking, wild temper, and tendency to spend what little money the family had on his habits "dominated and destroyed" the family.

"I hated that man ... still do."

Other than his mother's death from cancer, John reported few memories of her except that she was "nice" but always sick. His enduring memories of his mother involve spending most of his childhood days and nights caring for her as she grew more seriously ill.

When asked why and how the caretaker role fell to him at such a young age, John said, "Somebody had to do it. My sister left and the old man was a selfish drunk. I couldn't just let her die alone."

John grew up poor. The family managed to "get by" on what little money his father did not spend on alcohol and cigarettes. John's father took whatever work he could find but rarely spent his money on his family. John became even more impoverished when he moved in with his paternal grandmother, following his mother's death and his sister's marriage. His father did not want to take care of a 10-year-old boy, sending him to his grandmother's home permanently. Since that time, John has not contacted his father or siblings.

"Is your father still alive?"

"Don't know and don't care."

When asked about his education, John stated he had been a "good student" in high school. However, he dropped out in the 10th grade after being injured playing football and because his grandmother could not work anymore since she was sick and old. John began working full time to support his grandmother. She subsequently died a year later, leaving John alone in the world at 16 years old.

Within a year of dropping out and starting full time work, John earned his GED. After that, he enrolled in the local community college. John subsequently completed an associate degree and began working at his current employment. He had been there ever since. While claiming he was unhappy with his job because he was "always" passed over for promotion, he did not want to quit because he had seniority, decent pay, and "great" benefits.

As the end of our time together rapidly approached, I thought it was a good time to wind down. After thanking him for coming and participating, I assured John we could work on his marriage in the coming weeks. Since he said he was not planning to return home anytime soon, I believed the impending danger was mitigated, at least in the short term.

In this session, although demanding, I understood he did not have a drinking problem. I felt good we had an initial discussion about his drinking in relation to his marriage. I had a sense we had a long way to go on that subject in the future, assuming he returned.

"John, you want to schedule a session for next week?"

"Yeah, I guess so."

He appeared relieved now that our time was over. I was unsure if I would see him again.

QUESTIONS

The author assumed a nonconfrontational approach with John in the first session, being more concerned with relationship building than getting his entire story. Yet, many substance abuse practitioners believe a more direct, confrontational approach is required to help clients in denial about their substance use disorder come to grips with the extent of their problems.

This is more than a simple theoretical or style difference. The professional literature is producing a body of research that specifically addresses this difference and the role engagement and confrontation play in long-term treatment success. Therefore,

1. Explore the substance abuse and treatment literature looking for evidence of the efficacy of both nonconfrontational and confrontational approaches in substance use practice. Develop a position based on a balanced exploration of all sides of this argument.

At the end of the first session, John revealed important clues about his problems, experiences, and worldview. As you prepare for the second meeting,

1. Based on the information given in the first session, generate a preliminary list of John's problems and strengths.
2. What is your initial assessment? Write it down in a one-paragraph, narrative form like writing an article abstract. Come back to this and edit it after learning new information in each meeting.
3. What areas of John's life need further exploration? How do you plan to approach the issues when and if he returns?
4. At the end of the session, the author stated the imminent threat of domestic violence was mitigated because John was living out of the home. Based on your understanding and knowledge of domestic violence, how would you have handled this issue?

JOHN RETURNS

I wondered if John would return. When the appointed time arrived in the early afternoon, there he was, sitting in the waiting room. John seemed more relaxed this week, not as tense and unsure about what was to come.

In my experience, the first indication of potential client engagement happens when he or she shows up for a next session. I agree with Johnson (2004) that a first session is only successful if a client returns for a second. He implies that treatment begins when a client returns for a second session.

After exchanging social pleasantries and learning John and Lisa had daily interaction, but no altercations during the previous week, I decided to test our budding relationship by attempting to collect information about John's substance use history.

My goal for this session was to learn as much as possible about John's drinking history and habits. I wondered how he would react to my inquiry, since he was adamant about his lack of drinking issues in our first meeting. Once I learned he had no further negative or violent contact with Lisa in the previous week, I forged ahead, asking about his drinking history.

John said he drank for the first time at age 16, about the age he was left on his own after his grandmother's death and shortly before he met and married Lisa. He quickly added he believes he drinks "normally," especially compared to others in his family.

"My family is full of alcoholics—everybody but me," he claimed.

Of course, I learned earlier John's father had significant alcohol addiction issues, causing him to ignore and potentially abuse his family. According to John, it seems all the adult males, grandfather, father, and his three older male siblings all suffer with significant alcohol addiction. Apparently, John was the only adult male who managed to escape a significant alcohol use disorder … or did he?

Over the years I have come to expect clients to deny the existence of current substance use disorders. Many in the field believe the refusal to realize and/or admit to such issues is a function of denial or a refusal to admit problems to themselves. I have come to believe that denial is mostly a function of clients not wanting others, including family members, coworkers, friends, and especially practitioners to know that they, the client, know they have problems.

Experience has taught me there are usually several reasons for denial. First, as discussed earlier, substance use disorders carry a stigma and/or shame, shame of having lost control of their alcohol and other drug use, or being weak-willed, untrustworthy, and perhaps of being less of a person. It is naturally and psychologically protective for people to deny the existence of any issues or behavior for which they are ashamed. It is difficult for people to admit to this loss of control.

John appeared to be a man needing a sense of control over his life, as well as a person who experiences a great sense of shame and embarrassment about many things, including the violence in his marriage, his place in his church community, his upbringing, and his own ethnic heritage.

Second, if he were to freely admit what I suspected he already knew, that he was experiencing a significant substance use disorder, John had to assume responsibility and do something about it. He would immediately become accountable for his problems, his behavior, and the problems his substance use disorder caused in his life. Most people, including John, I assume, are unprepared for this realization and commitment, especially early in treatment. Clients will often readily admit to other problems, even more serious issues, rather than admit to a substance use disorder. For John, apparently, it was easier to admit to domestic violence, resulting in injury to his wife, than the possibility he might have a drinking problem.

As our discussion continued, John slowly admitted he drank daily, a significant change of story from our first meeting when he said he only drank "two to three times per week." He drank mostly beer, normally drinking 6 to 12 "beers" per day, capped off with three to four "shots" of vodka, mostly in the morning before work, and during the workday.

"How long have you been drinking like this, John?"

He pondered this question for a while, allowing the contemplative silence in the room to hang for what seemed like five minutes.

"I'd say I really began drinking more around the time Lisa had her accident," he said. "That was a really hard time for me. I thought for a while she was going to die or be paralyzed."

"What does drinking do for you?"

"It makes me relax, takes away my stress … lets me be calm and peaceful," he stated. "My life has been a mess for over 12 years. Having a few drinks every day is the only thing I have that's just mine, and it works, too."

"So, do 6 to 12 beers and a few shots of vodka make you intoxicated?"

"Nah, I can handle it. I don't really feel all that much of a buzz. I just feel good and normal is all."

"When is the last time you got really drunk?"

"Last weekend."

"How much did you drink last weekend?" I inquired.

"Probably a case of beer over the day and at least a pint of vodka … I took a drunk day for myself after all that happened at home. I deserved it."

"If you're going to get drunk, is that about how much it takes to get you there, normally?"

"Yeah, that's usually my weekends. I like to relax on weekends … but it's no problem for me. I deserve that time to myself."

Clearly, John's drinking patterns and amounts were different now from what he admitted to during our initial meeting. As we spent time together, he had obviously come to believe I could be trusted with his sensitive information. I find it humbling and a personal honor when clients begin trusting me as a person and professional. In this case, John had come a long way. But we were not done yet.

"John, have you ever tried to cut down or quit drinking in the past?"

"Yeah, I have. Lisa wanted me to quit a while back, so I did ... but after a couple days I decided she didn't have the right to demand that of me, so I gave it up and had a few drinks."

He went on to explain how he had "become" unable to ever relax on his own without drinking. When he did try to quit, John described what sounded like an overwhelming feeling of stress and anxiety. He even admitted feeling physically sick during those days, experiencing nausea, sweating, and headaches, along with significant anxiety. As if he knew what I was thinking, John quickly explained he must have been having a bad few days, and that what he just described was not related to alcohol withdrawal at all but likely the flu or a cold.

John also admitted he had accrued three drunken driving charges over the last 12 years. The first two occurred in years past, while he was presently awaiting trial on his third charge. He had been arrested some weeks earlier and found to have a .21 blood alcohol level (BAL) at the time of his arrest. In addition to trying to save his marriage, John also hoped that by voluntarily admitting himself for therapy, the courts might be lenient on him.

He dismissed his three arrests for drunken driving by claiming he was just "unlucky" and was being punished by "God." John also justified his record by claiming he knew many people who drank much more than he did who had not been arrested. Simply because he had been arrested three times for drinking-related offenses did not mean he was an alcoholic. He even asked whether I believed drunken driving laws were "too harsh." According to John, the law was to blame—not his drinking and driving. "I know people in high positions that drive under the influence all of the time. Some of them even get caught and do not get in trouble," he said.

John said he only drank and did not use any other drugs, except an "occasional" pain medication for his backaches. He experimented with marijuana when he was younger but claimed to have no interest in using drugs anymore. He said drinking "a little" allowed him to relax and have fun, and he did not need drugs. In John's mind, there was a clear distinction between "drugs" and alcohol, a common occurrence in substance use treatment.

It turns out this was John's second attempt at therapy. His first therapy experience occurred after one of his previous drunken driving charges. According to

John, therapy was an unpleasant experience primarily because he did not "need help," and he thought the therapist was an "idiot."

It was time for me to ask the big question. Although he had confided in me in ways I believed were honest, and our therapeutic relationship was off to a good start, this question and how I handled his answers could end it on the spot.

"Given what we discussed today ... have you ever wondered if you have a drinking problem?"

"NO! I don't drink any more than others I know, and besides, I've been doing this for years without a problem. I don't even get drunk when I drink, so it can't be a problem. My dad had problems, and I'm nothing like him."

John also said he did not have hobbies, except perhaps watching television and sometimes reading. He used to enjoy bowling and golf but had given up these activities over the years. He claimed he stopped these activities for no reason other than a lack of time. He denied that alcohol played a role in this change. For most clients when their substance use disorder increases, it begins to fill their free time and they begin letting go of hobbies and relationships where there is no substance use, and they begin to isolate.

"Taking care of Lisa and working became my full-time life."

Regarding his physical health, John claimed he was in good health. However, he also stated he sometimes suffered from backaches, headaches, stomachaches, and heartburn. When asked about the date of his last doctor's visit, John stated he did not "like doctors" and could not remember when he last had a physical examination. John believed his aches and pains, as he called them, were a normal part of "getting older."

His lack of medical care concerned me, especially because of his level of drinking. It is important to have clients obtain a physical health screening or complete physical examination if they have not had one in the last one to two years. Substance use and/or abstinence can severely complicate or exacerbate other health issues. For a client who is currently using substances or in the process of abstinence, practitioners must understand that physical, mental, and substance use disorders can mimic each other and exacerbate each other, sometimes becoming fatal.

Moreover, whether John admitted to an alcohol use disorder or not, his drinking history in terms of years of use, daily frequency, and amounts suggest that if he does decide to address it, he would need some form of professional and/or medical detoxification support. It can be physically and emotionally dangerous—to the point of death—for clients with a long history of heavy drinking or use of other depressant substances to stop cold turkey. The often-heavy withdrawal symptoms can lead to the exacerbation of underlying health issues, create physically threatening issues, lead to severe depressive symptoms, or trigger a heavy relapse that can lead to accidental overdose. Therefore, I recommend clients receive medically based detoxification services and not encourage them to quit on their own in isolation. Moreover, many clients are "medicating" significant co-occurring mental health disorders, making their diagnoses difficult while clients are using, since many mental health disorder symptoms mimic the symptoms of substance abuse and vice versa (Johnson, 2004). Hence, it is important for trained physicians to be involved early in the detoxification process in case a mental health crisis erupts once the substance abuse ends.

As our session ended, I thanked John for his honesty and willingness to talk to me about his life. John and I shook hands and scheduled an appointment for one week hence, knowing we were still a long journey away from approaching his substance use in a productive manner.

QUESTIONS

1. Now that we have a good look into John's drinking history and current use, check with the latest version of the *Diagnostic and Statistical Manual* (*DSM*) to see if you have enough information to decide upon a diagnosis.
2. If not, what further information do you need to make a confident diagnosis?

    Prochaska and DiClemente (1992) elaborate the Stages of Change model. We discussed this model in Chapter 1 of this text. Johnson (2004) uses the stages as indicators of a client's level of motivation. Based on your understanding of the stages of change:
3. At the conclusion of this session, what stage do you believe John is in related to his drinking? Defend your decision.

SESSION THREE AND BEYOND

John returned for a third session. In fact, I continued to see John as his therapist for more than one year. Below is a summary of John's life history. I gathered this information over the third and fourth sessions as I prepared a system-based assessment in preparation for successful treatment.

Mental Health Screening and Observations

During our first two sessions recounted above and over the following two weeks, John and I discussed other issues pertaining to his mental health status and well-being. I had to be careful with him during these discussions because John was sensitive to being labeled "mentally ill,' or, in his words, "crazy like that."

While I was not necessarily looking for mental illness, given that a high percentage of people with substance use disorders also have co-occurring mental health disorders, it was important to gather information to determine if a co-occurring mental health disorder existed.

My initial impressions of John from our early conversations, along with seeing and sensing his energy in my presence, left me with the belief that he was a rigid person, approaching his world in a dualistic manner. Things were either right or wrong; good or bad. John believed people were either with him or against him. John appeared unable or unwilling to see any middle ground. He was cognitively inflexible. For example, he was consistently unable or unwilling to appreciate or understand other people's perspectives if they differed from his, whether it was pertaining to me, his wife, friends, family, church friends, or coworkers. It was also apparent when he discussed immigrants, Mexican Americans, his heritage, or politics.

One of the most significant consequences of his "black or white" thinking was regular and sometimes intense interpersonal conflict. He argued and fought with nearly everybody in his life. He only seemed comfortable relating to people who agreed with him, saw their world the same way as John. If these people ever differed or changed their opinions, John saw this as a sign of disloyalty and a violation of trust. Thus, he ended the relationships.

There are many possible reasons for people seeing the world in this way. Often, people develop dualistic thinking to bring order and control in their lives; to reduce chaos and confusion. Whatever the reasoning behind such a worldview, this frequently leads people to be judgmental, rigid, intolerant, and stressed. Additionally, some people tend to adhere closely to certain rules and norms or values and find a correlation between this adherence and their self-esteem. This ego fragility when challenged can be expressed as high levels of anxiety, depression, or explosive anger.

John's life experience, including his abandonment by his mother and grandmother through death, his sister through marriage, and his father dumping him at his grandmother's, and the racial discrimination he faced by virtue of how he looked and sounded gave him a message of being devalued, unwanted, and/or unloved. This may have led him to cope by seeking self-worth through this dualistic approach to life, including his belief that he would rather be white than Mexican American.

John also found it difficult to see the "big picture" of life. He struggled to connect past to present, his environment to his daily life, or different aspects of his life to his overall well-being. He compartmentalized different domains of his life (i.e., marriage, drinking, mood, religion, etc.), talking as if these domains of his life were separate and did not interact. This is a common way of coping for many with substance use disorders, believing their use was separate from all the other difficulties in their lives (Johnson, 2004). It is also common for people to compartmentalize areas of life or behaviors that cause pain, stress, shame, or impact their self-esteem. This will often appear in session as client resistance, when it is really an indication of a primary, albeit dysfunctional, coping mechanism.

John presented as a man feeling pressure; the pressure to perform correctly in public and acting "right" in front of people. He seemed to try hard to minimize his anxiety. Most of the time, he seemed pleasant and friendly. However, he always had an "edge." His pleasantness did not seem genuine. He exuded an energy of seriousness and anxiety that permeated our session, making him seem ready to explode at any moment.

He desperately wanted the white majority to accept him as one of them. Unfortunately for John, I was not someone who could give him that sense of acceptance. As a Latino male, I was unable to provide those assurances for the long term. Yet, despite being suspicious of my background and apparently finding it difficult to trust me, John seemed to desperately want my reassurance that he was OK. He seemed to desperately want to convince people (and me) he was "right," "normal," and White. John had difficulty responding to questions about his life and how he was "doing" week to week, almost as if he were waiting for me to give him a clue about how he "should" be doing. He often asked me how I thought he was doing, looking for my approval of his actions. However, generally he dismissed my positive feedback. This behavior is not uncommon. It can be easy to forget the vulnerable position clients are in while receiving our services. The stigma of receiving such services, the associated low self-worth, and the need to be reassured they are okay often leads to constant approval seeking.

Paradoxically, these same people often seek and then reject our "approval" and care (unconditional positive regard) because trusting places them in a more vulnerable position. For many, our positive approach presents a contradiction to their negative worldview. Much of their life experience teaches people will ultimately hurt and reject them. Hence, for survival and self-protection, they reject us (and others) early as self-protection against the "inevitable."

Whenever I asked about his general feelings and mood day to day, he always said he was "good." Yet, minutes later he would talk about how he felt tense and restless most of the time; how these feelings made it difficult to concentrate. Later, John said he felt tense "all the time" because he "had" to always be right and good because "everybody" judged him.

Regarding his sleeping and eating habits, John reported having a generally poor appetite, and his sleep was sporadic, non-continuous, and rarely restful. Upon further investigation, John said his daily mood was often "blue." He said these feelings began as a child, becoming worse after his grandmother died but which escalated after his wife's car accident.

We needed to discover John's definition of feeling "blue," as there is no common understanding of what this means. It is always important to take the time necessary to discover a client's definition of words and not assume we know from our own personal or professional experience. John said feeling "blue" meant he often felt he was going through the motions, that nothing excited him or made him happy. He connected these feelings to his drinking, saying a few drinks "made" him relax and sleep better. He also agreed that his irritability impacted his interaction with others.

CASE SUMMARY

For this case, I presented John's personal information, taken from case records over five therapy sessions. At first, John seemed like a typical client with several complicated issues impacting his life. As is often the case, once I was able to gain John's trust, he allowed me to lead him on a joint exploration of his life, upbringing, and his issues and problems. We learned throughout this case that John's issues became intertwined to the point that they had to be addressed as concurrently as possible because each problem impacted and often exacerbated the others.

We discussed John's potential alcohol abuse and the upheaval and difficulties presently affecting his marriage. During that discussion, we also learned about his wife's car accident and her potential abuse of pain medications. Going further, we learned of at least one incidence of domestic violence and are left wondering whether his report of the last incident was the only event, or the tip of the iceberg between him and his wife Lisa.

Further, we were able to discuss his unsettled and often tumultuous upbringing with a violent and alcohol addicted father, as well as the significant loss he suffered throughout his childhood. Moreover, we discussed with John his potential mental health issues, along with his almost complete social isolation, paralleled by his overwhelming need to fit in and be accepted.

However, perhaps the most puzzling and difficult issue we learned about was John's commitment to distance himself from his Mexican American heritage—his keen desire to be seen as a member of the white majority and the lengths he has gone to not think of himself as a minority, a Latino, or a Mexican American.

We arrived at a point with John in therapy, where he needs a complete, multi-systems biopsychosocial assessment, complete with confirmed diagnostics of what appear to be multiple co-occurring disorders. He also needs to have a treatment that best suits his issues, strengths, and worldview.

This is where I leave the case to you for assessment and treatment planning. Good luck! Please begin by responding to the questions below. Use these questions, and the questions throughout the case, as a guide for your work planning to provide excellent treatment for John as his therapist.

QUESTIONS

1. To begin your work, please make a list of each diagnosis you have developed while reading this case. There will be at least one substance use disorder and at least one mental health disorder. Be prepared to defend your decisions by having client data to back up your decisions.
2. At the conclusion of this case, what stage do you believe John/Juan was in for each diagnosed problem?

ASSESSMENT, DIAGNOSES, AND TREATMENT PLANNING

Develop and write a comprehensive narrative assessment of John's life, family, and his environment. Your narrative assessment should reflect the information gleaned during his sessions. The narrative assessment includes a comprehensive diagnostic statement that integrates essential client information into a coherent description of their life, history, and current circumstances and concludes with the appropriate diagnosis (or, in this case, perhaps multiple diagnoses).

Once complete, use your findings from the narrative assessment and John's stage of change for each diagnosed problem to develop an initial treatment plan that can best address John's needs in the immediate future.

REFERENCES

American Psychiatric Association. (2013). *Diagnostic and statistical manual of mental disorders* (*DSM-5*®). Author.

Bridges, E. M. (2011). Racial identity development and psychological coping strategies of undergraduate and graduate African American males. *Journal of African American Males in Education, 2*(2).

Carlson, R. G. (2006). Ethnography and applied substance misuse research. In W. R. Miller & K. M. Carroll (Eds.), *Rethinking substance abuse: What the science shows, and what we should do about it*. Guilford Press.

Cross Jr., W. E. (1978). The Thomas and Cross models of psychological neuroscience: A review. *Journal of Black Psychology, 5*(1), 13–31.

DiClemente, C., Nidecker, M., & Bellack, A. S. (2008). Motivations and the stages of change among individuals with severe mental illness and substance use disorders. *Journal of Substance Abuse Treatment, 34*, 25–35.

DiClemente, C. C., & Velasquez, M. (2002). Motivational interviewing and the stages of change. In W. R. Miller & S. Rollnick (Eds.), *Motivational interviewing: Preparing people for change* (2nd ed.), pp. 201–216. Guilford Press.

Dunn, D. (2005). Substance abuse among nurses—defining the issue. *AORN Journal, 82*(4), 572–596.

Johnson, J. L. (2004). *Fundamentals of substance abuse practice*. Brooks/Cole.

Johnson, J. L. & Grant, G. (2005). *Casebook: Substance abuse*. Boston, Allyn & Bacon.

Helms, J. E. (1990). Womanist identity attitudes: An alternative to feminism in counseling theory and research. Unpublished manuscript.

Prochaska, J. O., & DiClemente, C. C. (1992). Stages of change in the modification of problem behaviors. In M. Hersen, R. M. Eisler, & P. M. Miller (Eds.), *Progress in behavior modification* (Vol. 28, pp. 183–218). Sycamore.

Room, R., Rehm, J., Trotter, I. I., Robert, T., Paglia, A., & Üstün, T. B. (2001). Cross-cultural views on stigma, valuation, parity, and societal values towards disability. In B. Üstün, S. Chatterji, J. E. Bickenbach, Trotter II, R. T., Room, R., Rehm, J., & Saxena, S. (Eds.), *Disability and culture: Universalism and diversity*, pp. 247–297. Hogrefe & Huber.

CHAPTER 4

Sara

Trauma, Mental Health, Substance Abuse, and Parental Rights

Carolyn Sutherby

INTRODUCTION

The case of Sara is complex and demonstrates the nexus between issues of mental health, substance use and abuse, and trauma in the life of a young woman in her twenties. This case involves multiple systems involvement with high stakes. For Sara, will she allow her past troubles and current problems to destroy what might be her last chance to have custody of her children? For her children, will Sara's inability or unwillingness to confront her past and present force them into a life growing up without their parent?

In the following case, I detail my interaction with Sara during a one-time, 90-minute clinical assessment interview. I withhold my clinical impressions, assessment, diagnoses, and recommendations to allow readers to explore—from a personal, theoretical, and legal perspective—what they would do in the same situation. If the readers are like me, these are the situations, with high stakes involved, that draw us to clinical practice with people experiencing co-occurring disorders.

SARA: CASE BACKGROUND

Sara's Child Protective Services (CPS) worker, concerned about Sara's mental health and substance use, referred her to my practice for a clinical assessment. I regularly receive referrals from the local sobriety/drug court and CPS, so I assumed Sara's case would be typical of other mothers I had worked with; women with trauma histories using drugs and alcohol to self medicate while living in poverty and being involved in unhealthy relationships. While I was right about some of these assumptions, it wouldn't take long to realize the unique nature of Sara's situation.

Described below is information I gained during our 90-minute initial assessment session. Typically, I reserve two sessions for information gathering and assessment activities. However, Sara's CPS worker requested my findings and recommendations about Sara's potential mental health and substance use disorders immediately so she could make some decisions about what would be in the best interest of her children. CPS opened Sara's case earlier in the week and sought my recommendations to guide their decisions about possible treatment options, preventive services, and other supportive resources. They needed to immediately determine if her children could safely remain in Sara's care or need to be removed for their safety and well-being. Fortunately, both Sara and I were able to accommodate a 90-minute session.

I hoped to gather enough information on which to base accurate diagnoses and make helpful follow-up recommendations. In an assessment session or sessions, it can be challenging to stay focused on these goals while still allowing clients to "tell their story." This is especially true when the referral source is asking for immediate, accurate, and helpful recommendations. If it worked out that Sara remained in therapy with me, I would have time to create a treatment plan with her to guide our clinical work and have time to dedicate to the therapeutic process. However, as of now, I was working on a one-session time limit. I hoped to be able to build enough rapport during that session to entice her to remain in therapy going forward.

I was encouraged to learn Sara volunteered to participate in our assessment. Generally, clients attending for assessment are mandated by CPS or a court order, making engagement, accurate diagnoses, and treatment planning difficult given their forced participation. Given the nature of my practice, I am used to meeting new clients who are unhappy to see me. While I try to avoid labeling these sometimes-hostile clients as "resistant" or "unmotivated," when it comes to their dealings with CPS or the court, these labels become real and are considered as part of court and child custody proceedings.

MEETING SARA

Sara showed up at my office about 10 minutes late for her appointment and remained talking on her telephone when I greeted her. She quickly apologized for being late, claiming her ride was late picking her up. They had also stopped at the store on the way to the session. She appeared well-kempt. Sara dressed in shorts and an oversized shirt and wore her dark hair in a loose, messy bun. Her neck and arms were covered by several large tattoos. She also had facial piercings in her nose, chin, and lip. She did not make eye contact, not unusual for a person meeting me in my professional office in the wake of a CPS complaint. Sara smelled of stale cigarette smoke.

I welcomed Sara into my office, and she accepted my offer for coffee. She found a seat in my overstuffed chair. We began by making small talk, designed to set a relaxed and conversational environment for our interview while she added multiple sugars to her coffee. I asked for her understanding of why she was referred for a clinical assessment.

"Why am I here … for you to decide if my drinking gets in the way of taking care of my boys."

"Do you think it gets in the way?"

Ignoring the drinking part of the question, Sara said, "You know, I'm a good mom … I love those boys more than anything and I know they are well taken care of, they have everything they need."

Sara signed a release of information so the CPS worker and I could communicate about her assessment. I took the time to explain that a copy of her assessment would go to the CPS worker, possibly her attorney, and the judge if her case went to court.

I further informed her I would be asking a lot of questions, some very personal, and if she wasn't comfortable answering she didn't have to. Finally, I let her know if I believed she presented a risk of harm to herself or others, I was forced to report this as well as any suspicion of child or adult abuse or neglect.

I believe it is important for practitioners to be mindful that we ask clients to be open and honest about their lives, knowing their stories often include reports of trauma, unsafe situations, drug and alcohol use, and mental health issues. It is challenging for clients to be honest with us, knowing that in situations like Sara's, people in positions of power will be interpreting her assessment and making decisions on her life based on the results.

Not only is this difficult for clients, but it is also important for practitioners to acknowledge the gravity of this process as well. What we see and decide can and will affect our clients' lives, and the lives of their children and other loved ones, perhaps forever. Hence, I always strive to be prepared, centered, and as open as I can be to ensure my assessment and recommendations are based on actual life circumstances, and not my interpretation of their lives or how I would prefer people to live. It is important to acknowledge these issues up front and validate the unique position in which it places clients and ourselves during these high-leverage clinical interviews.

Sara said she understood the expectations of the assessment and expressed interest in getting started. Her ride home would only wait for 90 minutes. After that, she'd have to walk home.

I immediately noticed Sara tapping her foot and bouncing her leg quickly. In addition, she chewed her fingernails. I've seen these behaviors in other clients who presented with issues involving substance use, ADD, anxiety, and trauma. It also could simply mean she was nervous. Instead of assuming what it all meant, I wanted to hear directly from Sara about her life experiences.

Sara is a 27-year-old white female in a relationship with the father (Mike) of her youngest child. She has three children: Luke, age 9; Jordan, age 6; and Blake, age two. Each boy has a different biological father and currently only Mike (Blake's father) is in the picture. Luke's father is incarcerated, serving a long prison term for drug trafficking. Sara has not had contact with Jordan's father since before he was born.

Sara currently resides with her boyfriend at his sister's house. Mike's sister has four children (ages 7–19) and her one-year-old granddaughter also lives in the home, along with "random people that come in and out." Sara wants to get her own place with Mike and her boys but understands this is challenging because they have little income.

Sara met Mike at a bar. She became pregnant with Blake the night they met. She said it was not what she would have planned but feels blessed to have Blake and thinks Mike is "a good guy." Mike has two other children Ariel (age 7) and Sasha (age 11). Mike rarely sees his daughters. Both girls live with their mothers, one in a different state and the other out of town. Sara said the child support he pays is "crazy, but he is mostly current on it." Sara has never received child support from Luke's or Jordan's fathers.

She is unemployed and currently trying to get approved for Social Security Disability Income because, according to Sara, her "panic attacks" are too severe for her to hold a job. She was denied Social Security "a couple of times before" but never appealed the decision. She plans to appeal this time if denied. For income, Sara works "under the table" for a friend's carpet cleaning business for the past year, but she only makes about $100 a month. Otherwise, she relies on her boyfriend for financial security.

Sara claims a high school diploma, no religious affiliation, English as her primary language, and she has no known or reported learning disabilities. She also claims she is not intoxicated or high from drugs at the time of the assessment. It can be difficult to know whether a client's self-reported sobriety is the truth. But if they are sober at the appointment, it is best to take their word for it until or unless their behavior proves otherwise.

CONTEXT OF HER REFERRAL FOR AN ASSESSMENT

CPS opened Sara's current case after she called 911 while intoxicated, claiming her neighbor was trying to kill her. When police arrived on the scene, Sara stood outside next to her car, while her son Blake was found sleeping inside the trunk.

When contacted by the police, she stated Blake was inside the trunk to keep him safe from her "crazy neighbor."

The neighbor admitted yelling at Sara to turn her music down. He claimed the interaction occurred after 1 am and he needed to sleep to be ready for work the next day. The neighbor denied threatening her.

According to the CPS worker at the time of referral, Sara eventually admitted she and Blake had slept in her car for a "few days" while her boyfriend Mike was out of town working. While client information can be helpful from a referral source, I prefer to hear my client's perspective on what occurred leading to a referral. It helps with relationship building when you make the client's opinions matter, instead of giving them the impression you already know their circumstances.

"So, Sara, what happened to get you involved with CPS?"

"I was drunk when I called the cops and really don't remember much. I think that neighbor guy is creepy, and he must have done something for me to need to protect Blake from him," she claimed.

"Anyways, CPS showed up because I guess they know my history. They let me and Blake stay with Mike's sister but now I have to follow a treatment plan to keep him and my other boys."

"What is in the treatment plan?"

"I don't know … I guess I'm supposed to come here … and oh yeah, not drink … and find a safe place to live."

Sara, Mike, and Blake had lived at a friend's house for the past few weeks after leaving his sister's house over an argument. They had to move from the friend's house because one of the homeowner's children bit Blake, making Sara feel unsafe in that home. She was planning to stay with her sister, but Helen's (her sister) boyfriend said no at the last minute.

"I didn't want to bother anybody else, so we slept in my car."

"What do you remember about your drinking that night? Were you alone with Blake the whole time?"

"I was drinking with friends most of the day and Blake was with my sister Helen. I don't know when she dropped him off, but I was going to stay with a friend, but his girlfriend came home and kicked me out. I think that's when I parked at my friend Shana's house and her neighbor started yelling at me."

"How did you get to Shana's from your other friend's house? Did you drive?"

"No, I would never drive drunk with Blake. Someone must have dropped us off with my car."

At this point, I had no reason to distrust Sara's account of not driving herself, but I made a note to revisit this if I could build a rapport with her. Further, she didn't seem to remember the evening, and I wondered if this was because she was in an alcohol-induced blackout, didn't trust me enough to be honest, or simply didn't remember.

This was Sara's third encounter with CPS. Both of her previous cases provided prevention services before being closed. However, her son Luke was placed in a temporary guardianship arrangement with his paternal grandmother, and Jordan now lives with Sara's maternal aunt, although not in an official guardianship. Each of these placements occurred because Sara was unable to provide her children a safe environment due to her alcohol and other drug use and lack of appropriate housing.

Sara told me it was her choice for the boys to live with relatives "until I can get my shit together ... then they will live with me again."

When asked how often she saw Luke and Jordan, Sara said it depended on whether she had a ride or her relative's "mood." "If they feel like letting me come over, they do; otherwise, I must talk to them on the phone. We talk every day."

SARA'S FAMILY HISTORY

Sara described her upbringing as "pretty normal." Her parents were never married. She was raised mostly by her mother (Cathy, a homemaker) until age 12 or 13. She saw her dad (Josh, a factory worker) mostly on weekends and holidays, but it wasn't consistent. She has no siblings from her parents.

Her mother married Dan, her stepfather, when Sara was four years old. They were later divorced when Sara was 13 or 14. Her mother and stepfather had a daughter together, and Dan had a son from a previous relationship. Presently, Cathy is in a five-year relationship with Phil. Sara gets along "okay" with her mom but finds her to be "judgmental."

Sara's biological father married when Sara was in the third or fourth grade. They remain married today. They have three children together: Ashley, Andrew, and Cory. Sara claims she gets along "okay" with her father and stepmother but always feels "like an outsider" and a "black sheep." Her parents both live in the same town where she grew up, but her siblings are scattered across the country. She has limited contact with her siblings except Helen and Ashley, whom she sees often.

When asked about abuse and neglect, domestic violence, or trauma while growing up, Sara responded, "Nothing like that ever happened at home, it was all later but not by my parents. They are good people."

She did not elaborate on this comment. Her body language and affect changed when I asked for clarification. She slouched down in her chair, avoided eye contact, and began wringing her hands. Instead of answering immediately, Sara first asked for more coffee with extra sugar. The prospects of talking about this, whatever it was, appeared to make Sara uncomfortable. I always want clients, especially new clients and particularly women with histories of trauma and/or abuse, to feel safe with me. To respond as if I am someone in whom they can trust with their stories and emotions. Hence, I decided Sara and I had not reached that moment. I was prepared to introduce her to some emotional grounding techniques if she became emotionally dysregulated.

MENTAL HEALTH HISTORY

When asked about her behavioral/mental health history, Sara responded with a laugh. "How much time do we have?"

Apparently, she was diagnosed with ADHD at age 8 and prescribed Ritalin. Sara claims she did not take it consistently.

"Do you know why you didn't take your Ritalin as prescribed?"

Pausing for a moment, Sara said, "Because my mom didn't think I needed it ... she said being hyper was my way of getting attention."

"Can you tell me more about your mom's opinion? Did she think you actually had ADHD?"

"Yeah, she knew I had ADHD ... I mean, I'm always losing stuff, I never can stay organized, and I get bored really easy. My mom always said I did things just to get attention and there was never really anything wrong with me ... like when I was cutting myself, she said I only did it to get people to notice me."

"Okay, we'll talk more about your cutting in a bit. What did your dad think about ADHD?"

"Oh, he didn't seem to care either way. He never really said anything, but my stepmom would always give me my pills when I was there. I think I was way too hyper for her. I stopped taking that stuff when I was about 12. I couldn't sleep or eat very well on it."

Sara says she began having symptoms of depression and anxiety in middle school but never told anyone and never received any treatment.

"What were your symptoms that made you think you had depression?"

"It was like not having any energy, feeling irritated all the time, not liking myself or how I looked, wanting to stay in bed, away from everybody all the time."

She continued. "My anxiety is the worst. I feel worried and scared all the time, I think people are talking about me or judging me, I can't stop thinking about problems to the point that I can't do anything else. I also have panic attacks where my chest hurts, my heart beats fast, and I feel like I'm going to die. My anxiety is all the time and depression is only a few times a month."

Sara said she currently experiences depression and anxiety symptoms and denied any inpatient psychiatric hospitalizations in her lifetime. She did see a therapist when CPS was involved before but didn't think counseling was helpful.

"I just went through the motions for court and didn't really want to get help ... I lied a lot to the lady."

Sara said she was now interested in therapy if she could see a woman who was not judgmental. To me, this was the beginning of positive signs for potential successful client engagement. However, she may be trying to manipulate me to help get a good report for CPS and the courts. Only time would tell for sure.

"Not now I don't ... but I tried to kill myself a bunch of times ... mostly when I was drunk. After high school, the first time, I took a bunch of this guy's pills that I was staying with. I woke up in a hospital and they said I was lucky to be alive, but I didn't feel lucky at all."

"Can you tell me about the first time you attempted suicide?"

"Yeah ... I just couldn't take it anymore and wanted to die. I'm glad I didn't die because now I have my boys, but it was crazy. I just had a bad few nights and was tired of all the craziness."

"Can you talk more about the 'craziness' that was going on?"

"No."

"Okay, that's fine. You said you attempted suicide a bunch of times; can you tell me more about that?"

"Basically, it would be when I was depressed and had been drinking. Once was after Luke was living with his grandma, I just didn't want to live without him. I took a bottle of pills ... but just fell asleep. My boyfriend said I was an idiot because I took melatonin but at the time, I really thought it would kill me."

"Any other times you can remember trying to kill yourself?"

"Only when I stayed in this one house. I thought about slitting my wrists, but I was too scared ... so I told my friend to give me a bunch of drugs so I would overdose. He said, why would I waste my stash so you can die?"

"So, did you do anything to try to kill yourself?"

"No, I just got super-wasted."

"Okay, do you remember any other times you have thought about killing yourself or made an attempt?"

"Probably another time, but I can't remember."

"Do you have any thoughts about killing yourself now? Or have you recently?"

"No, I don't want to die, I have my boys ... they would kill me if I did that (laughing)."

Sara denied any history of eating disorders, hallucinations/delusions, or other symptoms of bipolar disorder. She reports having a "normal" appetite but struggles with sleep. She claims she struggles falling asleep most nights, and when she does finally get to sleep, she wakes up several times and struggles to get back to bed.

Sara denied having any self-harming behaviors. "Yeah, I used to cut on my arms (shows therapist marks on her inner forearms), but that was a long time ago. I haven't done that shit in years."

"When do you think was the last time you cut your arms?"

"High school."

"Did you cut anywhere else on your body? Or try other forms of self-harm such as burning, pulling out hair?"

"No, I only cut my arms."

"When you cut on your arms, were you doing that to attempt suicide?"

"No, I liked to feel the pain. It was a relief, I guess."

"Okay, so the cutting on your arms and times you tried to kill yourself were different, is that right?"

"Yeah."

"With everything that has been going on, have you had any thoughts of cutting?"

"Not really, I mean no. I don't think it would be a good idea. No, I don't."

FAMILY MENTAL HEALTH HISTORY

Sara says she does not believe her parents were ever treated for mental health or substance use issues. She did say here paternal grandpa "was a total alcoholic and died from it."

"My mom has anxiety, she just won't talk about it ... she is wound so tight all the time, and everything always has to be perfect. People can say what they want about me being on meds and stuff, but my mom needs something to calm her down for sure."

"Has anyone else in your family ever attempted or died from suicide that you know of?"

"No, I don't think anyone has even tried ... but I don't know anything really about my siblings."

MEDICAL AND MEDICATION HISTORY

Sara says she is "sick all the time" with stomach and back pain. She was in a car accident in her late teens and said this "messed up my back really bad." She had her gallbladder removed at age 25 and reports having three "normal" labor and deliveries for her children. She denied experiencing any postpartum anxiety or depression after the births of her sons.

"How many pregnancies have you had?"

"I have three sons. That's all you need to know about."

"Okay, I won't ask about it then. What about your stomach pain?

"I think it's due to stress ... I think I might have had some ulcers that were never treated. I also have ovarian cysts that flare up but nothing else medical."

She could not remember her last medical appointment or physical examination. Nor could she recall anything about her own child development history other than "my mom said I was a really hard baby."

Sara said she has taken "every kind of medication to treat anxiety and depression" but couldn't remember names, dosages, or prescribers other than Zoloft and Xanax, her current prescription. Sara doesn't think her meds are working and wants to talk to her doctor about changing them.

"Have you found that self-medicating for your depression and anxiety or pain issues helps?"

"You mean like weed?"

"Yes, or other substances."

"Weed really helps my anxiety and pain. I got my card, but CPS still won't let me use it. I don't think I ever used anything else ... well, maybe alcohol and drugs to numb the pain."

"When you think about using Xanax or weed, which helps with your anxiety more?"

"Oh, boy, I guess if it's really good weed, that works, but sometimes, I get too paranoid on it ... so probably Xanax, but they don't give me enough. I need more than what they give me to really help."

"What about treating your physical pain? What has worked the best?"

"I hate to say it, but Oxys (OxyContin) and Percs (Percocet) help with my pain the best, but they are hard to get nowadays. I try to take hot baths or watch what I eat ... also watch my stress, but it's hard now with my situation to not get stressed." (Sara begins crying.)

"It seems like you have a lot going on to feel stressed about ..."

(still crying) "Yeah ... no one understands how hard it is. Mike is always pissed at me, my older boys are gone, CPS is up my ass ... it's like nothing I do seems to be enough."

"It sounds very difficult."

"You don't know the half of it."

"I'd like to know as much as you are comfortable telling me."

My efforts at being supportive seemed to be working, until she appeared to hit an emotional and/or trust wall. Her posture and affect changed abruptly.

"Whatever ... I'm fine, let's keep going. I know there are more questions."

"Yes, I do have more questions, but if you start to feel upset, we can always take a break. I know it is difficult to talk about some of the things you have experienced. Do you think we could practice a grounding technique so if you start to get uncomfortable, you'll know how to relax while you are here today?"

No longer crying, she responded curtly, "Sounds good."

I talked Sara through a simple breathing exercise to help her relax and stay in the present moment. She said she liked the practice and it helped her to relax. After she calmed, I explained trauma and gave some examples such as car accidents, medical diagnosis, sexual or physical assaults, domestic violence. She said she understood what trauma was and admitted she did experience "lots of trauma" but didn't want to talk about it.

I wanted to get a more accurate picture of her trauma history but in a way that did not make her feel threatened or retraumatized. I like to use the PTSD Screen PCL–Civilian Version. It is an easy, nonthreatening series of questions most clients are willing to answer.

"That's okay. I'd like to ask if you have ever experienced any of the following things from this list I have here. Is that okay with you?"

"Sure."

Sara scored over 5 on the PTSD Screen PCL-C.

QUESTIONS

1. Look up the PTSD PCL–Civilian Version screening instrument to determine the meaning of Sara's score of 5 on the scale. It is in the public domain and available for use.
2. Explore other trauma screening instruments that may best suit your practice and practice preparation.
3. It is also helpful to become familiar with the Adverse Childhood Experiences Scale (ACES), also readily available in the public domain.

"Based on the way you answered these questions, Sara, it seems like you have a lot of symptoms of trauma. Lots of people don't know that what they are feeling can be a result of the trauma they endured. Many women I work with don't understand how trauma can cause certain physical and emotional symptoms, even if it happened years ago."

She paused, appearing to give my words some thought.

"I guess I never thought about it like that. I do have a lot of bad dreams, and I'm always worried about what will happen to my boys ... Mike says I'm overprotective. I kind of think I deserve to feel this way though because of everything I've done. If I feel normal, it doesn't seem fair ..."

"Tell me more about why it isn't fair."

"Everybody has bad stuff happen to them, I'm no different, except I did bad stuff to other people, so why should I feel okay. I have made it this far in life. I'm a good mom, but I know what I did, and I deserve this."

"So, you think because you hurt other people that you deserve to feel hurt yourself?"

"Yes ... definitely. Just so you know, I never hurt my boys. This was a long time ago."

"That's a heavy burden to carry. How long have you felt this way?"

"I don't know, awhile. I guess since high school ..."

"You've mentioned high school a few times today ..."

"Yeah, it was crazy. I think that's really when things got crazy."

The first time she mentioned "things got crazy," she abruptly refused to discuss it. When she said it again, I believed she was signaling she might be ready.

"What do you mean by crazy?"

"When I started getting more into drugs and stuff ... partying a lot, not caring about anything or anyone. I joined a band, we sucked (laughs), but yeah, it got crazy."

SUBSTANCE USE HISTORY

"Well, since you mentioned drugs, now is probably a good time to talk about your substance use history. Can you start with when you first drank alcohol and tell me about how your use progressed?"

"I think I was 12 or 13 when I first drank ... it was beer from an older neighbor. We were at a block party or something I don't remember, but I didn't really think about it. He just said do you want some, and I drank it. After that I didn't really drink again for a while, I would've probably but didn't really have an opportunity. When I met Dustin is when I started drinking regularly, I must have been 15 or so ..."

Sara said her alcohol use went from drinking beer with her boyfriend Dustin and their friends on the weekends to "all day, every day" by the time she was 16. Sara claims drinking "made me feel like I fit in. I was smart, funny, beautiful, and really happy." Most of her friends drank the same as her—"to get drunk"—and her typical amount of alcohol at one time was a 24-pack of beer split with a couple of friends and a pint of liquor. She drank after school and on the weekends but occasionally drank before and during school.

At 16 years old, Sara dropped out of high school and was secretly living in Dustin's basement for almost two months until she was arrested for shoplifting and placed in juvenile detention. She was transferred to a rehabilitation program for substance use disorders where she stayed for 30 days. Upon discharge, she moved in with her mom and stayed sober for nearly a year. She returned to school and eventually graduated.

"Dustin hooked up with my best friend while I was locked up, and that really messed me up. I pretended I was okay, but that's when I first cut on my arm. I think that replaced drinking for a while."

"Did you use any other substances besides alcohol during this time?"

"I smoked cigarettes and tried weed a few times, but I liked alcohol. I didn't get into drugs until the summer after I graduated. That's when I met Sam."

"Okay, before we talk about that, can you tell me about your experience in rehab and staying sober?"

"Rehab was dumb; it was a bunch of other kids in trouble with the law. I didn't think I was an alcoholic and really heard crazy stories and figured I would keep drinking when I got home, but Dustin broke up with me and my mom threatened to lock me up longer if I didn't graduate, so I just chilled for a while. It wasn't hard to not drink."

"What changed? Why did you drink again?"

"I stared hanging out with people who drank again and fell right back into it."

"So, who is Sam?"

Sara met Samantha (Sam) at a restaurant where they both worked the summer after she graduated. Sam was 21. At first, Sara thought she was "cool" because she was in a band, had her own place, and had interesting friends. They quickly began a sexual relationship, but Sara kept this hidden from her friends and family, afraid of what they would think of her.

One night after Sara had been drinking heavily, Sam asked her to have sex with one of her male friends for money. Sara doesn't remember much about it but reports this soon became a familiar pattern—Sam convincing her to sleep with men she arranged for money.

"It really wasn't that bad. Most guys were nice, and I started singing in the band and we made a lot of money. I didn't really think it was a big deal."

Sara moved in with her bandmates and continued drinking heavily. She began having alcohol-induced blackouts and started to miss work with hangovers or because she "didn't care." Over the next few years, her alcohol intake increased to a 30-pack of beer and pint of rum each day. She would get shaky and experience nausea if she didn't drink.

One night at a bar, a woman told Sara that Sam was "pimping her out" to make money. Sara also learned that night Sam had been sleeping with a lot of other women, also convincing them to have sex with men for money. Sara says the news really hurt her, and she proceeded to get "really wasted" that night. Later that night, she was arrested on her way home and charged with a DUI. She remained in jail for two days until her dad bailed her out. She doesn't remember driving home or being arrested.

"Before you share the rest of your substance use story, could you tell me about your legal history? Any other arrests or charges besides the shoplifting and DUI?"

"Yeah, I have three DUIs total and a prostitution charge. I've been off probation for a while now but still don't have my license back."

"Okay, so you don't have any current criminal charges and aren't on probation?"

"Nope, I'm all good now, but I think if I get another DUI, I could go to prison."

"What can you tell me about your prostitution charge?"

"It seems obvious, don't it? I got picked up for prostitution. It was my first offense, so I was only in jail a few days. It was stupid, but I needed the money for rent, so whatever."

I asked Sara how often she had to prostitute herself for the money to meet her basic needs.

"Oh ... every once in a while, but it's been a few years." She denied ever sleeping with someone for alcohol and/or drugs or for money to buy alcohol and drugs.

"Can you tell me about your drug use history? I think I only know about smoking marijuana a few times."

"Yeah, so I kept drinking, but honestly, I started getting sick a lot from it, and a friend of mine said weed was better because I wouldn't get sick, so I started smoking every day. I was talking to Sam again, and she didn't like weed, so I had to hide it. But eventually when I got into the business side of things, I had to slow down the weed."

"What do you mean, the business side of things?"

"I don't really want to talk about it now ... but let's just say I stopped being the one sleeping with guys, but still got paid."

"Okay, so you were working with Sam, not for her?"

"Sort of. (She curls up into the chair, crosses her arms, and avoids eye contact.) I never thought about it as a job. It's hard to talk about. I just didn't want to sleep with any more dudes, but the money was so good ... I don't want to say anything more."

"I can tell this is difficult to talk about."

"Yeah, so, back to the drugs (laughs). I had Luke by this time, and his dad was the one who introduced me to dust (PCP). I loved it the first time I used it, but my man got busted so my supply ran out (laughs). After that, I got into OxyContin and Percocet (both opioid drugs) and went back to drinking. I was mixing vodka and diet Coke, that was my favorite, or just plain vodka."

"What about heroin?"

"No ... I basically tried every drug you can imagine other than that. Coke, LSD, 'shrooms, meth, ecstasy, Special K, I don't know all of them ... but somehow not heroin."

"What would you say is your drug of choice?"

"Well, alcohol is my go-to, but as they say, I don't discriminate—if something is around, I'll try it. I do really like the combination of vodka and dust the best, it's the best high for me. At my most, I was drinking a half gallon of vodka every few days."

"When was the last time you used any substances?"

"No drugs for a while, I guess a couple of weeks ... but I'm still drinking."

"You said you weren't drunk or high when we started this assessment, but did you drink today?"

"Not yet (laughs). I don't feel good, so I know I will probably need to have a drink after this, but I'm sure CPS says I can't drink at all, so I'm going to cut back at least. My mom said I needed detox because of how much I can drink, but I haven't been getting sick or having the shakes or whatever, so I'll just drink less and see how that goes."

"Okay, I know CPS has said you need to stop using alcohol and drugs, but what do you think? Do you see yourself as someone with an addiction? If not, then how would you describe it?"

"I don't know if I'd label myself an addict. I mean, I don't live under a bridge drinking out of a paper bag or anything. I work, take care of my kids, and I don't see how CPS has the right to say how I live my life."

"At the beginning of the assessment, you said you should cut back on your use. What does that look like to you?"

"I think CPS is stupid, my kids' lives aren't in danger, but they deserve to have a stable home and stuff. A good mom wouldn't put them in this position. I mean, they aren't even living together. Brothers should live together, and it's my fault. I know that CPS has the power to decide if I keep my kids, so I should have known better than to be back in this position."

"Okay, what about your drug and alcohol use?"

"I can stop using drugs, no problem. And if CPS makes me stop drinking, I will, if it means getting my kids all back."

"Have you tried stopping before?"

"Yeah, when CPS made me a while ago. I just think it's stupid that someone else can decide if my drinking is a problem. Shouldn't that be my decision? If I really thought I couldn't take care of my kids or go to work because of my use … I would say so."

"How did you stop before? Did you go to meetings, work with a therapist, cut back slowly, or all at once?"

"They made me go to AA and NA meetings, but they didn't help. I did meet some nice women, but as far as stopping, it was up to me to do it, no one else. I was clean for 6 or 7 months until I got the boys back. Then I started drinking again, so that's why the older boys aren't with me now."

"So, you said if you couldn't take care of your kids because of your drinking you'd stop, and Luke and Jordan cannot live with you now because of your drinking. What does that mean to you?"

"It was my choice to let them stay there. CPS didn't make me."

"What about the night that the police were called, and Blake was in the trunk? You don't seem to remember much about that night."

"Look ... I trust myself and know that I put him in there because he needed to be safe. My gut was in charge, and it told me what to do. I know how to survive, believe me!"

"What about sleeping in the car, do you think this was a safe situation for Blake?"

"Yeah, he was safe. He was with me all the time, it's not cold out, and we had food and stuff. We are in a house now, and when Mike gets back with his check and if my disability goes through, we'll have enough money to get our own place."

Sara seemed unable or unwilling to connect the impact of her substance use and the current troubles in her life, including her new CPS case and this interview. This was apparent in her lack of insight about how her substance use affected her ability to parent and/or her legal authority to be a parent. I believe she loves her boys and seems genuine when claiming it was her choice to place her older boys to live with relatives. However, her reality seems distorted, since she is not willing or able to recognize this choice was made in part because of her substance use and pressure from CPS and the courts.

Our 90-minute session time grew short. I typically close these sessions by asking if there was anything I forgot to ask or what else she thought I needed to know before we ended. She talked about how much she loved her boys and that she would do "whatever it took" to make sure they could all live with her again. She also said she would be willing to come back for individual therapy with me.

"Does 'doing whatever it takes' mean if you have to stop using alcohol or drugs, would this be possible, and if so how?"

Sara was quiet for a long time. "I still don't think I should have to stop drinking."

I validated her attitude of not being "told what to do" regarding her drinking or parenting, for that matter. I asked whether she could reframe the idea of CPS making her stop drinking to focus on her desire to be the best mom possible. That is, can she learn to take CPS out of the equation and think about whether drugs and alcohol interfere with being a great mom?

"Yes ... I can try. I do often feel tired and irritable after drinking a lot, and this makes me snap at the boys sometimes."

"On a scale of 1–10, with 1 being "low" and 10 being "high," where do you place your willingness to stop using alcohol and other drugs?"

"Oh ... probably a 4 or 5."

"What would it take to increase that number to a 7 or 8?"

"I don't know ... probably if CPS says I have to stop. I don't want them to take Blake away from me."

"You know, Sara, this could be an opportunity for you to learn about whether your substance use is serving you in a way that makes your life better, or just helping you survive emotionally. I can tell that you love your children, and it says a lot that you came today, something you didn't have to do."

"Thanks ... I do love my kids. I just want them back."

"If you did decide to quit, since you've been using alcohol and drugs for so long, it would be difficult to stop without having a strong support system, a realistic plan, and coping skills to replace the substances, and you really will need to be medically detoxed for your own health and safety."

"You've been doing the best you can with what you know for a long time. Hopefully, therapy could help you learn new skills and ways to manage your stress, depression/anxiety, and trauma symptoms without relying on drugs and alcohol. You've had periods of sobriety before, so it is possible. We just need to figure out how to make this your decision rather than CPS's."

Sara did not respond. But she did appear to be giving my words serious thought. Perhaps this was a beginning; perhaps not. At least she appeared to be thinking about it.

"What do your think are the biggest barriers to meeting the expectations laid out by CPS?"

"Transportation. We have a car but no insurance, and I have a suspended license and shouldn't be driving at all. We also have little money, so finding housing we can afford will be really hard."

At the end of an assessment, I try to be as transparent as possible with clients in terms of diagnosis and recommendations. For instance, if a client presents with criteria for major depression and I'm recommending weekly individual therapy and a psychotropic medication review with their physician, I tell them before they leave. I also tell them if I need some time to review my notes before making a formal diagnosis.

I thanked Sara for coming and being honest about her life. I wished her well, and said I hoped to see her again soon. We shook hands, and Sara walked out.

CASE COMMENTS

Sara was referred for an assessment after falling under the auspices of Child Protective Services (CPS) a third time. She was found sleeping in her car while apparently intoxicated, with her young son Blake asleep in the trunk of the car late at night. Sara, a 27-year-old White female, presented an interesting and sometimes tragic life story, complete with years of trauma-related issues, mental health issues, medication use, sex trafficking, and alcohol and other drug use and abuse.

She presented for this voluntary interview under the guidance of her CPS worker for an assessment, diagnoses, and treatment plan as part of CPS determining her fitness to remain in custody of her two youngest children. While CPS does not have to take the recommendations from this session, normally these recommendations become part of the legal requirements for maintaining parental rights.

Performing assessments of this type brings with its significant responsibility for practitioners, as these recommendations can and will affect the future of children, beyond that of the adult parent.

We ask readers to place themselves "in my shoes" as the professional handling this case. As readers, you have all the information I had when this session ended. Other than seeing her in person, which is valuable, of course, you know everything I knew when I had to write my assessment, complete with multiple diagnoses, and a treatment plan that considers all relevant information contained in the interview.

I purposely omitted my thoughts, assumptions, and conclusions so as not to bias your assessment in any way. These are the kinds of clinical situations, persons with multiple co-occurring diagnoses with difficult-to-assess levels of motivation, that most pursuing careers in clinical practice seek. Adding to the difficulty, in these situations often, our decisions will have long-term, life-changing effects on everyone involved. That is, Sara, her children, potential caretakers, and others have everything at stake. These are the situations we sign up for in this profession. Good luck as you work through the details of this case while developing a professional assessment, diagnoses, and treatment plans and recommendations for Sara and her future.

QUESTIONS

1. **Further Information.** What questions did the author leave out of the assessment?
    - What would you have done differently throughout the assessment?
    - Are there questions you would not have asked or pushed for more information on?
2. **Develop a Genogram.** Based on the case information in this chapter, develop a three-generation genogram (also including important non-family members if needed) to represent Sara's presented life and all who are instrumentally involved. Make any notes and figures on this genogram to aid in developing a holistic view of this case.
3. **Issues and Strengths List.** Make a list, with supporting evidence, of the main issues in Sara's life at the time of the interview. Include a list of Sara's personal and social strengths that may be used as resources in the future pertaining to each of the issues listed.
4. **Narrative Assessment and Diagnoses.** Develop and write a narrative assessment and diagnosis(es) as demonstrated by the information contained in this case. Justify your diagnostic decisions by listing the criteria you believe are met through the interview record. It is inappropriate to base diagnostic decisions on assumptions; use only direct evidence provided by your client.

- If you met Sara, what additional information would you need to contribute to a more comprehensive narrative assessment and diagnostic decisions?
- Be sure to place Sara's personal and social strengths in the narrative assessment, to be used later as part of treatment planning.

5. **Stages of Change.** As discussed in Chapter 1, here is where we initially apply the stages of change (Prochaska & DiClemente, 1992; DiClemente & Prochaska, 1998) developed to assess the client's motivation for change for each diagnosed problem (Johnson, 2004).
   - List each diagnosis you decided upon in the narrative assessment for both substance use and mental health disorders.
   - For each diagnosis listed above, determine what stage of change Sara is presently in pertaining to her motivation to change that problem. Please use Sara's own words to justify your stage decisions.
   - Use the stages of change during the next section on treatment planning.

6. **Treatment Plan.** Based on the narrative assessment, develop a written treatment plan to include short- and long-term treatment goals and objectives. Include what methods of treatment and support you will utilize.
   - What treatment theory or combination of theories do you believe best fits Sara's reality? Defend your decision.
   - What theories or approaches does the latest empirical evidence in the field recommend?
   - Based on the stages of change decisions in Question 4, where will you begin in treatment? Explain and defend your decisions.
   - Pertaining to treating people with co-occurring disorders, what do the current professional literature and practice evidence suggest as the most effective way to proceed when it comes to deciding which issues to treat first?

7. **Intervention Planning.** Based on the treatment theory or theories chosen and defended above, list each intervention you would use in your work with Sara. Specifically, for each intervention, include the target issue, intervention, and modality (i.e., group therapy) you chose and the theoretical justification for each.
   - What other options might be available should these interventions prove ineffective?
   - What does the latest empirical evidence in the field suggest for each target issue? How does this evidence match with your intervention strategies?

- When developing treatment approaches, do not overlook nontraditional approaches and approaches that target multiple systemic levels (i.e., individual, family, community, advocacy, etc.).
- What factors and strategies will you use to build trust and engagement during the intervention phases of your work? How will you assist Sara as her motivation to change waxes and wanes over the coming weeks and months?
- What if her personal goals do not align with yours? For instance, if she says she wants to focus her sessions on healthier communication with her boyfriend rather than issues surrounding her mental health or substance use.
- Think about the initial therapy session after the assessment with Sara. How would you begin, what would your goals be for the session, and what would you hope to accomplish?

8. **CPS Recommendations.** Based on the information provided by Sara, what would you recommend to CPS regarding Sara's ability to keep Blake safe in her care? Be sure to align any recommendations with the diagnoses you decided for Sara above.
    - Do you think she can remain his primary caretaker?
    - If she is capable, recommend any services needed for her to have a chance to succeed.
    - If she isn't capable, why not? What are your reasons for coming to this decision?

REFERENCES

DiClemente, C. C., & Prochaska, J. O. (1998). Toward a comprehensive, transtheoretical model of change: Stages of change and addictive behaviors. In W. R. Miller & N. Heather (Eds.), *Treating addictive behaviors* (2nd ed., pp. 3–24). Plenum Press.

Johnson, J. L. (2004). *Fundamentals of substance abuse practice.* Thomson-Brooks/Cole.

Prochaska, J. O., & DiClemente, C. C. (1992). Stages of change in the modification of problem behaviors. In M. Herzen, R. M. Eisler, & P. M. Miller (Eds.), *Progress in behavior modification* (Vol. 28, pp. 183–218). Sycamore.

CHAPTER 5

Appearances Can Be Deceiving
The Case of Mark Johnson

Salvador Lopez-Arias and Jerry L. Johnson

INTRODUCTION

Human beings are prone to believing in stereotypes. We look at someone, hear about their personal "success" and often look at their race and/or ethnicity and come to conclusions about their life and how it must be for them compared to others. Clinical practitioners, as human beings first, are not immune to this problem. While in daily life, believing a stereotype to be true probably does not matter as much, in clinical practice, it is misguided, often dangerous, and even unethical, depending on one's professional code of ethics.

When it pertains to people with co-occurring disorders, unless one is careful, it is "easy" to prejudge who these people are, what they look like, and how financially successful they can be given their problems and issues. Words come to mind like *junkie*, *drunk*, and *dope fiend*, each conjuring a negative picture and image of who most people are who have co-occurring disorders. As clinical practitioners, it is our professional task to overcome our humanness, in that we must find ways to move beyond the normal, and find ways to set aside our personal beliefs, biases, and life experience. That is our job, and it is one that will last throughout one's career. No level of experience or number of clients makes us immune to falling into the trap of stereotype and our own subjective ideas about people and their problems, backgrounds, upbringings, and histories.

The case presented in here, Mark Johnson, is a case that may challenge one's perceptions and stereotypes about just who are the people who come to therapy with significant co-occurring disorders.

Mark Johnson, a Harvard-educated, former college athlete, wealthy businessowner in the financial services sector, and apparently popular man does not "look" the part of a troubled client with a troubling background. In fact, he looks the opposite. He appears at an outpatient clinic in his home city for an assessment after being arrested for Driving While Intoxicated (DWI). He wears an expensive business suit to the first session, claiming the whole arrest "thing" is a waste of his time; the police stopped and arrested him because they were jealous of his success, as is everyone else. Mark comes across initially as the epitome of an adult White male, loaded with a sense of entitlement and privilege, ready to use it at any cost to get out of trouble. Besides, he is successful and White—how troubled can he be? As experienced practitioners learn, it is important to approach every client, regardless of appearances and income statements, as unique people from unique backgrounds and avoid the human tendency to assume … oh, it must be a mistake. He cannot be that successful with that many problems. Or can he?

We present Mark Johnson's case differently from the cases in previous chapters. In the preceding cases, authors took readers inside the actual sessions to hear some of the dialogue and understand the process of data collection and motivation, to allow readers to read what the experienced practitioners were thinking and planning as the sessions proceeded. It's almost as if our authors/practitioners were thinking out loud during their cases.

In this chapter, instead of being inside the sessions, we present a completed Client Assessment form that includes all of the personal information and data collected during the assessment process. Following assessment protocol, each completed section of this assessment form contains data, along with relevant personal quotes from the client. However, the sections are devoid of "clinical assessment thinking." That is, we have omitted the practitioner's thinking, conclusions, diagnostics, final assessment report, and treatment plan.

It is for the readers to read the case assessment report, and complete each section based on the information contained in the client data. At the end of each section of the assessment form, there is a place to write concluding paragraphs called "Issues to Consider" and "Strengths to Consider." Readers should complete these sections under each assessment dimension before moving to the end of chapter tasks.

After completing the Issues and Strengths sections throughout the chapter, at the end of the case, there are five important areas to be completed, either alone, in groups, or as a class. These sections include:

1. Clinical Diagnoses: Readers will use the client information to make clinical diagnoses. There will be at least one substance use disorder and at least one mental health disorder. There may, in fact, be more.
2. Stages of Change: Readers will determine the relevant stage of change for each clinical diagnosis, along with the justification for said change (see Chapter 1 for more on the Stages of Change).
3. Narrative Assessment: Readers will write a complete narrative assessment, encompassing all client data, including clinical hypotheses and conclusions. This narrative must be holistic and be consistent with the clinical diagnoses made earlier (Johnson, 2004).

4. Treatment Plan: Using the information from above in combination with knowledge of treatment modalities, intensities, and methods, develop a treatment plan for Mark moving forward. The treatment plan will include treatment goals, measurable objectives, and a rationale for each section.
5. High-Risk Aftercare and Intervention Plan: Based on Mark's presentation and life circumstances, here you decide how his case will be handled in the event of any high-risk activities and behaviors and how these will be handled by the professionals and through recommendations or referrals for the client.

It is important to remember that all assessment and clinical conclusions, diagnoses, and decision making must be based on data contained in the case. That is, while it may be appropriate to speculate about issues based on new information learned later in therapy, any documented conclusions must have data to back them up. Conclusions without data represent the practitioner's implicit or explicit bias, out-of-control subjectivity, too much reliance on personal life experience, or simply overconfidence (Johnson, 2004). Please take steps to help avoid making clinical decisions based on practitioner life experience, beliefs, attitudes, and thoughts. This exercise is good practice about an issue that professionals must be aware of throughout their clinical careers.

Mark Johnson is an interesting case for study. Good luck with this case.

SUBSTANCE ABUSE ASSESSMENT

Guide for use: Each dimension requires data, narrative, and a short summary of the relevant issues and strengths to consider in the final assessment.

Client Name: Mark Johnson   Date of 1st Contact: 00/00/00

Clinician: Date Completed: 00/00/00

Client description, presenting problem, and context of referral

A. Brief Description of Client

Mark Johnson presents as a 49-year-old, multiracial male (Native American/White). Mark appears in good physical condition, and his dress is appropriate for both setting and weather. He is dressed in a business suit, since the appointment occurred during the business day. This is congruent with his profession as the co-owner of a financial services business. Mark self-identifies as a heterosexual male with "many girlfriends," which appears to make him proud. Mark graduated from Harvard University with a bachelor's degree in finance. He also played football at Harvard. Mark currently owns his own investment business with one business partner. He claims his business is "very successful."

B. Chief Complaint and Symptoms by Client and Others Present

Mark indicates his "only" reason for attending this assessment is because of his recent legal troubles involving an arrest for Driving While Intoxicated (DWI). The arrest, his third overall, occurred two weeks prior to the assessment. Mark denies having a substance abuse problem, stating that he "drinks responsibly." He further says that he's not interested in therapy because "therapy is for weak people." Mark does not appear interested in any talk of drinking problems but did seem interested in talking about his "depressed moods," "nervousness," and a 30-year pattern of suicidal thoughts and gestures, beginning at 18 years old. Throughout the session, Mark repeatedly said he is not an "alcoholic" and only drinks responsibly.

Mark's chief complaint is law enforcement. He believes they wrongfully charged him with DWI, and that he "was not drunk at all." He claimed he was being victimized by law enforcement, who were "jealous" of his obvious success in life. "They took one look at my BMW and decided it was my turn to be taken down." He went on to say that he "knew people in this town" and that it was a matter of time before "this whole thing went away."

C. Context of the Referral, Precipitating Events, Facts, and Dates

Mark's attorney referred him for this assessment. Mark claimed he "hated" therapy and counseling and had no express interest in participating. Further, he said that therapy and counseling were only for "weak-minded people."

At the time of his arrest, Mark was leaving a Hollywood-themed party at a local bar. He originally called it an actual Hollywood party, later changing it to a Hollywood-themed party. As he drove toward his house, the police pulled him over for failure to maintain his driving lane. The police noticed he smelled of alcohol and was having trouble word finding, so they ordered him out of his vehicle and administered a series of field sobriety tests, including a Breathalyzer.

Initially, Mark said he "blew" a .098 on the Breathalyzer test (over the .08 BAL limit in his state). He later revised his statement to say he "actually blew a .14." This BAL put him near his state's "Super Drunk" violation, which carries harsher and longer-term penalties. He also failed the field sobriety tests. His reason for failing the sobriety tests was he missed dinner that day and was "worn out from playing volleyball" before going to the party. Mark insisted the Breathalyzer had to be wrong because "I wasn't even buzzing at the time."

When he was arrested, Mark had several friends in the vehicle. He was angry because the police "humiliated" him in front of his friends, two of whom were professional clients of his investment/financial planning business. Mark emphatically stated he "wasn't drunk" and was "driving just fine." Mark believes the police were stationed outside the bar and pulled him over because "they wanted to take down someone in a Beemer." He compared his arrest in his town to a "celebrity takedown." "Getting someone like me is a score" in the eyes of the police. According to Mark, this was his third arrest for DWI in the last ten years. He received probation and was assigned to attend drunk-driving education classes as punishment for his first two offenses.

While he clearly stated his dislike for therapy and therapists, Mark was willing to answer questions about his history, current life, and behavior. He did not present as someone who was angry, hostile, or resistant to the assessment process. He seemed deeply convinced he was correct, normal, and that law enforcement was out to get him.

Issues to Consider in Assessment (Complete Section Based on Data Presented Above):

Strengths to Consider in Treatment (Complete Section Based on Data Above):

Treatment History

A. Substance Abuse Treatment (Self and Family Members)
Mark claims he has never participated in substance abuse assessment, treatment, therapy, or counseling. He was mandated to attend "drunk-driving classes" twice in the past as part of legal requirements after his first two DWI arrests. Mark claims his uncle "went to rehab" twice and his father twice. He said rehab was a "waste of time" for both because neither quit drinking and both were still "assholes" when they were done. He insists he does not need counseling, therapy, or rehabilitation for his substance use.

B. Client Attitude Toward Substance Abuse Treatment

Mark is against participating in treatment; mainly, it appears he does not believe he needs it. He stated that "rehab is for weak people" and "if you have a problem that you want to stop, you should just stop." Mark is only attending this assessment at the request of his lawyer and claims he has no need or interest in counseling or therapy beyond his legal proceedings. "If this helps me stay out of jail, ... then okay." He stated that he was sure treatment was good for some people—"you know, drunks and junkies and people like that"—but he certainly (in his mind) is not one of "those people." He wondered aloud how anybody could think he was a drunk or a junkie, given all the money he makes and the beautiful house and cars he owns. He does not appear to be resistant to treatment; he does not think it applies to him at the time of the assessment.

C. Mental Health Treatment (Self and Family Members)

Mark claims his parents "made" him see a psychiatrist as a child (around age 12) for depression, nervousness, and what he called his "acting out ... being loud, fighting, being generally hard to handle." He said he "hated" his "weirdo psychiatrist" and "the only thing he did was give me medicine to try to calm me down." He claimed, "I never took it."

Since then Mark says he has not received any other mental health treatment. "I'm not crazy," was his stated reason for not having or needing mental health treatment.

As an adult, his family physician began prescribing an antidepressant medication because of his complaint of being "down" and "nervous" much of the time, along with intermittent bouts of anger and rage, often ending in him getting into bar fights. However, because the medicine came from his long-time family doctor, it wasn't for being "crazy," but for feeling "ill."

D. Attitudes About Mental Health Treatment(s)

Mark says his antidepressant medication he was prescribed as a child made him feel "dead." He stopped taking "whatever it was" and lied to his parents and doctor. "I threw them away and told my parents and the doctor I was taking them."

In adulthood, he has always taken his antidepressants, even though the meds often affect his sexual performance. However, he also believes the antidepressant medication seemed to enhance the effects of alcohol. Mark states the antidepressants do not help his mood much, but he has kept taking them in any event.

His attitude overall about treatment for mental health is not different from substance abuse treatment. He does not believe he needs it; hence, he says he does not want it. Not resistant so much as disinterested.

Issues to Consider (Complete Section Based on Data Presented Above):

Strengths to Consider (Complete Data Based on Data Presented Above):

Substance Use History

A. Lifetime Substance Use History

SUBSTANCE	FREQUENCY	Dose (avg.)	Age 1st use	Age last use	Route of Admin.	Overdose
Alcohol	5–7 times per week					
Marijuana	3–4 times per month	Unknown	15	49	Smoke	No
Percocet	Unknown	Unknown	34	49	Oral	No
Morphine	Unknown	Unknown	Early 20s	Early 20s	Oral	No
Vicodin	Unknown	Unknown	Early 20s	Early 20s	Oral	No
Mushrooms	2–3 times	Unknown	Late teens	Early 20s	Oral	No

*Data in table discussed directly below.

B. Drugs Used in Previous 30 Days

According to the Substance Use History chart above, Mark reports drinking an average of eight drinks per day, five to seven days per week. He estimates he has consumed this much alcohol daily for "as long as I can remember." He also admitted to smoking marijuana at least once per week on average and taking Percocet (opioid painkiller) daily during the previous 30 days. During the session, Mark said he drank daily in the previous week, smoked marijuana twice, and took his pain medication "three to four" times per day for pain treatment. Mark was vague when asked if he took his Percocet according to the stated doses on the prescription.

Mark said he sometimes takes a drink in the morning as an "eye-opener" and he would drink occasional shots at work to help him maintain his "focus." Mark denied these morning drinks helped ward off withdrawal symptoms and said it does not mean he has a drinking problem.

C. Drugs of Choice

Mark said he prefers alcohol, marijuana, and Percocet. He claims to have tried other drugs, but the combination of these three drugs "takes care" of him well, including his attitude, mood, and pain level. He claims to have lingering knee and hip pain from his days as a football player, and the Percocet "takes care of it very well." He said he drinks for energy and to "party" and smokes "weed" to mellow out and relax. Often, his marijuana use is later at night as he prepares to relax and sleep. He prefers bourbon, whiskey, beer, and "expensive wines."

D. Drug Mixing

Mark claims he often uses alcohol and marijuana at the same time and claims he "mixes" different types of alcohol together; while he prefers bourbon and whiskey, he says "I'm not picky." Typically, Mark says he uses marijuana to "mellow out" and alcohol to "party."

Mark did not mention the daily mixing of alcohol (a depressant drug that slows the central nervous system) and Percocet (an opioid painkiller combining oxycodone and acetaminophen). This drug combination has been part of his daily intake, according to the substance use table, for the previous 15 years. He also did not mention his daily mixing of alcohol in relatively large amounts with Percocet and daily antidepressant medication.

E. Longest Period of Abstinence

Mark reported that he refrained from alcohol use for a period 20-plus years earlier during college while being treated with morphine and Vicodin to overcome multiple knee surgeries. He said the university doctors required he not use alcohol with those opioid drugs. When asked, Mark claims that Percocet is "different" from what he took in college, so he does not worry about it.

More recently, two years prior to this session, Mark abstained from alcohol use for four days when his girlfriend asked him to participate in Lent at her church. Mark stated that he experienced flu-like symptoms during this period, including feeling "shaky," having a headache, upset stomach, and nausea. Mark was adamant these were not symptoms of alcohol withdrawal. He claims he had the flu during the same four days. He also said he continued smoking marijuana and taking his pain medication during that time, each of which would have made his physical symptoms from not drinking less intense. He had a few drinks at midnight of the fourth day. He said this was the only time he had been without drinking for more than one day since he was in college.

F. Narrative (Include Attitudes and Beliefs, Use Patterns, and Symptoms That May Support or Refute Any Substance Use Disorder Diagnoses)
Mark reported he first began drinking alcohol and smoking marijuana at age 14 (35 years earlier). Mark's report of the dosage and frequency of his alcohol use varied slightly throughout the assessment process, but consistently said he drank five to seven times per week, going back at least 25 years to his college days. Sometimes, Mark would claim he drank less, but this appeared to be in relation to his sense that I was concerned about his use. Eventually, his reports would align consistently with the more frequent five to seven days per week.

Initially, Mark reported drinking 10–12 drinks per day, but later reduced this to approximately eight drinks (either shots, mixed drinks, or beer). Mark claims he drinks because he "loves" it; it helps him relax; soothes his nervousness and anxiety; and seems to lessen his symptoms of depression. He claims he typically drinks with friends during the week and weekends, and it is an integral part of all his various social activities. He says he does drink shots throughout his workdays to help him feel "focused" and that he sometimes adds bourbon to his morning coffee as an "eye-opener." Mark states he frequently engages in physical altercations with strangers in bars and at parties while drinking but claims it is not because he's drunk, but because the "world is full of assholes." He also reports that after drinking, he notices that sometimes his depression symptoms increase, but marijuana seems to help with that.

Mark says his drinking and smoking as a 14-year-old was the same as all kids, "drink some here and there on weekends after football games, smoke a little weed here and there ... stuff like that." His drinking increased after he left home, but not by much. In college, he had a serious girlfriend and had boundaries placed on his behavior by being a scholarship athlete, which he claims kept his drinking and partying to a minimum.

However, things changed for Mark when he was a sophomore. His girlfriend, the "love of my life," was killed in a single-vehicle car accident, one in which Mark was driving. He said it was a slippery night in the northeast, and he lost control of the car on a curve and flew off the road into a ditch. The car flipped and rolled, and his girlfriend was ejected and killed. Mark's injuries were minor. He said he blamed himself for her death and has experienced "survivor's guilt" almost every day since, including dreams and nightmares about her and the event continuing to the present day. He was not charged by law enforcement. Her death was ruled accidental.

Mark said the aftermath of the accident is when his drinking increased, gradually approaching the levels of drinking he reports presently. He claims drinking helped his guilt early on after the accident, and then "just sort of remained part of my life … no problem … just part of who I am." He again reported current dreams and nightmares about the accident that continue to the present day. He also said he still "gets nervous" driving on ice-covered roads and occasionally gets déjà vu when he is out in those conditions.

Mark says he is in "complete control" of his drinking, can quit or cut down at any time, and as proof of his control claims he "never" gets "wasted," only "buzzed." Mark says he chooses when to drink and is not controlled by any urge to drink. He says he is responsible for his drinking, as evidenced by always knowing what he is doing, not getting "sloppy," not waking up with a stranger, most always remembering how he got home, and winning any fights he gets into at the bar.

Mark defines being out of control as stumbling around, being an "asshole" at the bar, not remembering how he got hurt, spending a large amount of money without remembering it, and passing out. Mark stated that the last time he drank in an uncontrollable manner was five years earlier, although he used to regularly drink in this manner when he was younger in the months following the fatal accident.

About his multiple DWI arrests, he states that "everybody drinks and drives," including friends and family members. He seems to believe his multiple arrests had little to do with his drinking and driving and more to do with bad luck, being in the wrong place at the wrong time, and police jealousy. Mark said he was always "in control" each time he was pulled over, and he previously "blew" BAL levels of .09 and .15. He claims that even a .15 BAL (nearly twice the legal limit) did not make him feel intoxicated. He received probation and education for each of his earlier arrests.

Mark adamantly claims that neither he nor his friends believe he has a drinking problem and that "I drink less than a lot of people, including my friends." Mark mentioned two emergency hospitalizations for alcohol overdose, but he says these happened because somebody "spiked" his drinks, not because he drank too much.

Currently, Mark's driver's license is suspended. He is allowed to drive only to and from work and therapy until his case is determined in court. Mark says this case will work out in his favor because he has "pull" and the resources to hire a great attorney. "Only poor people go to jail for this petty shit," he claimed.

The only person in Mark's life who has ever asked him to watch his drinking is his best friend and business partner, Joe. Mark claims Joe has asked him not to drink during business dinners with clients or accept alcohol from customers in their homes. While he continues to drink occasionally at work, he masks his use with Joe during these meetings. Because of this tension with Joe, Mark indicated he has been trying to cut down on his drinking during the workday, with marginal success.

Mark reports using marijuana when he wants to "mellow out" and sometimes while doing other activities such as hiking with friends. Mark indicates that he rarely mixes alcohol and marijuana (although the substance use chart says otherwise) but will if he is already drinking and is offered some. Mark claims marijuana "takes the edge off," especially at night before sleeping. He also reports it helps when he feels "down," better than alcohol sometimes.

As stated earlier, Mark has a "standing" prescription for Percocet, originally to treat the long-term lingering effects of serious knee and hip injuries/surgeries from his college football career. He began using Percocet in his mid-30s after realizing that over-the-counter pain medications did not work. He was vague about his prescribed dose compared to his use but says it has "never been a problem" and that he does often enjoy the enhanced "mellow buzz" he believes his "Percs" and alcohol provides.

Regarding other lifetime substance use, Mark reports previously using mushrooms, morphine, and Vicodin. Mark reports using mushrooms in his late teens and early 20s but hasn't used them since as he didn't like being out of control. The morphine and Vicodin usage was due to the football injury and subsequent surgery Mark underwent during college. Looking at the themes of his substance use chart, it appears he prefers drugs from the depressant categories, as he reports no incidence of the use of stimulant drugs in his lifetime.

Issues to Consider (Complete Section Based on Data Presented Above):

Strengths to Consider (Complete Section Based on Data Presented Above):

Medical History

A. Health Issues

Mark indicates that he sustained significant injuries to both knees and his left hip while playing college football at Harvard. This led to multiple surgeries and several months of opioid medication. He continues to experience "a lot of pain" at the time of this assessment, for which he has been taking Percocet daily since he was 35 years old (14 years total). He reported no other significant injuries or illnesses since that time.

B. Health Treatment and Current and Past Medication

Mark said he has yearly physical examinations, and just completed that within three months of this interview. He claims he was healthy, and there were no serious medical issues. He claims his doctor performs routine blood work. Mark was found to have elevated blood pressure and cholesterol. He claims he refused medication, claiming, "I'm too young for that ... I'll be fine." He said his doctor does not test for alcohol and/or other drugs, nor does he focus on liver or kidney function. Mark became angry at what he assumed was my suggestion that his alcohol use could be causing liver or kidney damage.

Mark previously took antidepressants as a child (refused to take them) and has been taking a prescribed antidepressant for nearly 20 years as an adult. While he says it helps "some" with his mood and nervousness/anxiety, Mark claims that it helps enhance the effect of alcohol, so he continues to take it. Mark was hospitalized twice while drinking, although he indicates that this was not connected to alcohol but that he thinks someone "spiked" his drinks, because he is never that out of control.

Issues to Consider (Complete Based on Data Presented Above):

Strengths to Consider (Complete Based on Data Presented Above):

Basic Needs

It appears Mark currently and comfortably meets his basic needs for food, clothing, and shelter. Mark claims he co-owns an investment business that provides a "significant income." He says he owns his own home in an upscale neighborhood and drives several cars, including his BMW that he claims made the police "jealous." Mark does report consistently driving while under the influence of alcohol, which may endanger his personal safety as well as the safety of others. He claims no financial problems but did mention he carries significant personal debt (credit cards, loans, mortgage, cars, etc.).

Issues to Consider (Complete Based on Data Presented Above):

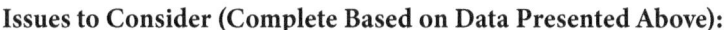

Strengths to Consider (Complete Based on Data Presented Above):

Mental Health, Psychological and Emotional Functioning

General Appearance

1. **Physical appearance:** Mark's physical appearance was neat and clean, consistent with his age and stated social class position and income.
2. **Attitude:** Mark's attitude appeared to change between friendly and cooperative to negative, suspicious, bordering on angry, and hostile. He does appear preoccupied with his "wealth" and position as it relates to others and their attitude toward him. He was open in the assessment session, seeming not to care what I or anyone else thought about his behaviors. He also spoke a lot about his need to be in control.

Behavioral Functioning

1. **Motor activity:** His level of motor activity seemed normal and appropriate for the context of the assessment. He was able to sit still and focus on the issues at hand, without much motor activity associated with nerves or anxiety.
2. **Gait:** His gait appeared normal and steady.
3. **Posture:** His posture appeared normal. He made good eye contact and had a firm handshake.
4. **Speech:** Mark's speech and speech patterns appeared normal for the circumstances.

Emotional Functioning

1. **Mood:** Mark discussed having bouts of depression and anxiety over the course of his lifetime for which he was medically treated, as he is currently. In this session, he also appeared anxious, although some of that could be related specifically to the purpose of our meeting. His mood fluctuated during the session from anxious, to angry, to withdrawn and quiet but seemed to sense this and came back to a more anxious presentation. He was open to discussing his problems with mood and seems to have conscious knowledge of the potential self-medicating behavior provided by his alcohol, marijuana, and Percocet use. His mood darkened when he discussed the death of his girlfriend in an accident where he was the driver over 30 years ago, in some ways reflecting someone discussing a more recent tragedy. As stated earlier, Mark reported current dreams and nightmares about the accident that continue to the present day. He also said he still "gets nervous" driving on ice-covered roads and occasionally gets déjà vu when he is out in those conditions.
2. **Affect:** His affect was appropriate to the session. He spoke with confidence and seemed to be concerned about showing himself as successful, smart, confident, and in control. His affect did become flat when discussing the auto accident described earlier.

    Thought process:

    Mark's thought process appeared appropriate and normal on the surface; however, he did report frequent bouts of suicidal ideas and thoughts that have led to attempts on his part.

    Thought content:

    Mark appears to be invested in presenting himself as smart, together, confident, and in control. Yet, he also appears to have highly self-critical thoughts while presenting as highly confident. He seems measured and planful in his thinking, ensuring he presents himself in the "correct" manner to match his external self-image needs.

He discussed several bouts with suicidal ideation and planful, if not impulsive, attempts at suicide. He also appears to be unable to balance evidence of issues in his life (i.e., arrests for DWI, feeling sick when not drinking, etc.) to his behavior. His need for control and notions that the police (and others) are jealous of his status driving them to act against him is another area of concern.

Perceptions:
Mark experiences no evidence of perceptual problems or issues.

Cognitive Functions:

1. **Consciousness:** Mark was alert and appropriate.
2. **Orientation:** His orientation to time, place, and person was normal.
3. **Memory:** His memory was normal for past and present.
4. **Attention/Concentration:** He appeared to have normal ability to concentrate and remain focused.
5. **Intellectual function:** He is an intelligent person with an excellent vocabulary and was able to complete thoughts and follow the conversation, even apparently able to sense when certain questions in the assessment had larger meaning or connections (i.e., liver screen medical question).
6. **Insight:** Mark's insight is poor across several issues in his life.
7. **Judgment:** Mark's judgement is poor as demonstrated by his high level of alcohol use over time, his drug mixing, suicide ideation and gestures, and continuously driving under the influence despite legal troubles. Moreover, he continues to drink at work while telling his partner he does not and likes to get in fights at bars.

Mental Health Status, Psychological and Emotional Function Narrative

Mark was cooperative, although somewhat suspicious and guarded during the interview. Still, he discussed all topics identified. Many of Mark's answers were frank and defensive. Mark presented as relaxed and indifferent by laughing and rationalizing his substance use behavior.

Mark reported no current behavioral problems. He did indicate he engages in altercations and fighting while at a bar, indicating that he is typically the person initiating these events. He only wants to fight men who are being "jerks" toward women. Mark indicated he starts these fights when he is feeling "down" to release frustration. Mark stated that as a child, he would get into fights and break things to help him to feel better. As noted above, Mark's motor activity, gait, and posture all appeared normal.

Mark's speech was normal, and he was quick to answer most questions and topics presented. Mark's speech was very fluid and spontaneous throughout the session.

Mark's affect presented as appropriate throughout the assessment sessions. Mark's mood was anxious during the initial session as evidenced by his spontaneous responses and nervous mannerisms. At other times during the session, depending on the topic being discussed, Mark's mood presented as depressed and sullen. This was especially true when he discussed the death of his girlfriend 30 years ago. Mark said he consistently felt "blue" a couple of times per week. He stated that it feels like the depression he experienced as a child. Mark indicated his sadness typically occurs when he feels like he cannot do anything to help others or himself with problems, making him feel out of control. He stated that "no one can be happy all the time" and sometimes wonders "is this all there is to life."

Mark said he experiences insomnia, which he copes with by smoking marijuana, drinking, and medication use. He attributed some sleep problems to the dreams and nightmares he continues to have over the accident.

He copes with the depressive symptoms by spending time with friends and girlfriends as well as drinking, which only makes the depression worse if he drinks too much. Mark indicated that he does not want to talk to a professional about his depression as he is "not sad enough to require therapy" and "not crazy enough to see a therapist."

Mark reports current, frequent thoughts of suicide that typically occur multiple times per week. He has a stated history of suicide attempts and gestures. He claims he has often "wanted to die" since childhood but did not try to kill himself as a child.

Mark says he first tried suicide at 18 when his girlfriend died suddenly in a car accident, where he was the driver. Frequently ("probably ten times"), Mark has driven his car at high speeds through the city, hoping to lose control and crash or get in an accident and die. He also reported current dreams and nightmares about the accident that continue to the present day. He also said he still "gets nervous" driving on ice-covered roads and occasionally gets déjà vu when he is out in those conditions.

In adulthood, he acts out his suicidal thoughts by playing Russian roulette with his personal revolver. He claims he pulled the trigger "three times" with no result before he stopped. He says he has played Russian roulette at least five times in recent years. Recently, after his last DWI arrest, he claims to have driven his BMW at speeds in excess of 100 MPH through a winding part of a local expressway in hopes of crashing. He said he "chickened out" when he heard his tires begin squealing.

Mark said he decided he did not to kill himself that night because he did not want to "go to hell," "become a vegetable," or hurt others. "If I'm going to do it … I want to make sure I die and not become disabled." Presently, Mark said he has no solid suicide plan and describes the nature of his thoughts as "What if I did this or that to die?" He claims to have these thoughts most every day. His attitude toward suicidal thoughts is that "Everyone thinks about killing themselves."

Mark identifies the cause of both his depressed moods and suicidal thoughts as more likely during times he is unable to solve his own problems, making him feel out of control. He also said he feels the worst when he gets thinking about his deceased girlfriend after being triggered during the day or going through a period of frequent dreams about the accident.

He says he owns several firearms, including handguns and long guns for hunting. Mark indicated that he owns guns for hunting which he would never use for suicidal or homicidal purposes, despite having engaged in Russian roulette.

Mark's thought process is appropriate and easy to follow. His thought content is typically appropriate, although suicidal thoughts are present. Many of Mark's thoughts tend to be preoccupied with being in control and ensuring people see him as rich, smart, attractive, and successful. At other times, Mark seems to be preoccupied with suicide, his deceased girlfriend, and mood stabilizing.

Mark's cognitive functions are normal. He reports no hallucinations, is alert, and is oriented to time, place, and person. Mark's memory appears normal as does his level of attention, concentration, general knowledge, and intellectual function.

Mark's behaviors and statements indicate that his insight and judgment about his substance abuse are poor. Mark indicated that he drinks to relax as well as to party but also uses it as a mechanism for coping with his depressive symptoms. Mark also rationalized his withdrawal symptoms, claiming his symptoms were due to the flu. Although Mark states that he is a "responsible drinker," he states that "everyone drinks and drives" and regularly participates in this type of behavior.

He also indicated that he felt in control and not too intoxicated to drive when he was pulled over the most recent time as well as in the past. Mark has maintained that he is trying to cut down on his drinking due to input from his business partner, which shows improving insight and judgment. Finally, his lack of insight about the potential dangers of regularly mixing alcohol and opioid pain medication is concerning.

Mark's developmental history is normal. His motor, language, and cognitive skills developed normally. Mark reports that he did very well in college and described himself as athletic and "got good grades," although he did not speak much about his performance or experience in school while a child or adolescent.

Mark reports that he has no history of a learning disability. He was in his family home until he was 17 years old when he moved out to escape physical and mental abuse by his father and grandfather. Shortly after that event, Mark's first girlfriend died in an accident. Mark indicated that it was this event that led to an increase in his drinking as well as suicidal ideations and behaviors. This also appears to be the time where Mark's apparent mood issues were exacerbated.

Issues to Consider (Complete Based on Data Presented Above):

Strengths to Consider (Complete Based on Data Presented Above):

Family History

Mark grew up in a two-parent household with three younger brothers in a middle-class, close-knit neighborhood north of town. Mark's father worked in a factory and his mother stayed at home. As a child, Mark claims he was always blamed for his brothers' misbehavior and was punished by his father when they did not behave. He also indicated that he often saw his father "pushing" and "slapping" his mother "a lot" during his childhood. He says his father was an abusive man; he "always yelled and hit me and everybody else."

At the age of 17, Mark moved out of his family home after a fistfight with his father. He said he could not take it anymore. He moved in with a family friend in order to complete high school. Mark also claims both he and his siblings were verbally and physically abused by his paternal grandfather until he left home. He has always felt like he let his family down because he left, while his mother and siblings had to stay in that abusive household and family.

Mark's parents and siblings moved to Florida 20 years ago; his grandparents still live nearby in nursing homes. Mark does not visit or talk to them because of the past.

Mark currently talks to his mother regularly, but she always "bugs him about getting married and having kids." He stated that while he was growing up, "the only one that cared was Mom." Mark does not talk to his father, stating that "he's an asshole, a horrible human being." Mark also has little communication with his brothers as they have never been close and "they still kiss my Dad's ass, and I don't." Mark claims his father must have "worn them down" over the years, but he "couldn't do that to me." He also stated that he is not close to his brothers as they "get drunk" at family gatherings and "I'm not into that."

Mark's mother has a college degree in nursing and his father dropped out of high school around the 11th grade. His mother began staying home when she became pregnant with Mark, which is why she married his father. Mark reports that he has a bachelor's degree from Harvard University in finance. When asked how he was able to go to such a prestigious institution after he left home at an early age, Mark became defensive and proud while discussing how he did it all by himself with academic and athletic scholarships.

Mark reports the police were called several times to the Johnson home over his father's domestic violence against his mother. Several times the father left for short periods, but "Mom would always take that bastard back." He claims he vowed he would never treat a woman badly.

As stated above, Mark reports a long history of physical and verbal abuse as a child. He states that his father was always "yelling and hitting" both him and his mother. Mark recounted the event that caused him to leave home at 17 years old. At a family birthday party, his younger brothers were drinking and his father became angry, accusing them of making a fool of him. Mark's mother responded, "Well, look at their example." Mark's father pushed his mother, and Mark physically intervened. Mark's father had to go to the hospital due to injuries sustained in this altercation. Mark also stated that "I remember abuse my whole life."

Mark also reports physical and verbal abuse from his grandfather, claiming they would yell, pinch, pull his ears, and threaten to spank him with a belt. He also states they were always angry. Mark reports no history of sexual abuse, although he did discuss sexual relationships with older women while he was a young teenager.

Mark reports no history of diagnosed mental health issues, although substance abuse issues were prevalent in his family. Mark described his father as an alcoholic who "stumbles around and fights at family events." He states his mother "drank until she found Jesus." Mark also indicated his brothers drink often and to excess in irresponsible manners. He discussed drinking being present at all family gatherings as well as how he remembers going out with family members and "getting plastered." It is also commonplace for members of Mark's family to drive while intoxicated. Mark also indicated his grandfathers were always drinking, although he never saw them drunk, so he doesn't think they were alcoholics. Mark maintained that two of his uncles received substance abuse treatment but were unsuccessful. Other than these two family members, Mark was only able to identify one other family member who does not drink to excess.

Issues to Consider (Complete Based on Data Presented Above):

Strengths to Consider (Complete Based on Data Presented Above):

Cultural/Spiritual Context (Racial Identity, Oppression/Discrimination)

Mark identifies as "American," although he states that he is multicultural, including Native American and White. He also identifies as nonreligious, although he does believe in a higher power and has attended church at the request of his girlfriends. He did state that he is not sure this higher power has ever looked after him, especially since the deadly accident. "Not sure how a loving God could let that happen."

Mark also said he has not followed through with his suicidal attempts due to a fear of "going to hell."

Issues to Consider (Complete Based on Data Presented Above):

Strengths to Consider (Complete Based on Data Presented Above):

Social-Relational and Social Support

Mark's only reported "committed" relationship was with his first girlfriend. He was 17 years old and she was 25. He stated they spent lots of time together; she was the only person he could talk to; he would do anything for her; she "showed me lots of stuff"; she took him out of his shell; they went on trips; and he has never felt the same with anyone else. When describing himself in the relationship, Mark indicates he was like a "lost puppy" as he would do whatever she wanted. Interestingly, he flashed some anger when saying that about himself. They dated for one year until he was 18 years old. As stated earlier, she was killed in a single-car crash while Mark was driving. He claims to believe she was his best chance at love, that they were meant to be together.

After her death, Mark began exhibiting more risky behaviors, including driving fast in hopes of being hit or crashing, suicide thoughts and gestures, drinking heavily, using drugs, and having multiple, superficial sexual relationships with women. He claims it took him a "few years" to get over her loss and the guilt associated with being the driver, losing control of the car, and surviving the crash. He has not been in a committed relationship with a woman since.

Currently, Mark says he has many female friends who all know about one another. Mark stated that his friends come and go, with the longest one staying for two years, although he is still friends will all of them. He indicates he is in sexual relationships with each, and they all enjoy recreational activities together. He typically spends time with one female friend at a time but insists the four or five others understand the nature of the relationships. Mark also indicated his friends help him cope with his depression as they are always around for support. He claims to have closer relationships with two women who are more "special" than the others to whom he can talk about his sadness.

Mark maintains that he also has male friends he likes but does not spend as much time with them. He claims his recreational interests include driving, outdoor activities, exercise, camping, boating (he made sure to tell me how "big and expensive" his boat was), and going to the bar. Mark says his friends do not think he has a substance abuse problem as they all drink the same as he does. He states his friends tend to expect him to "pay for stuff" since he makes more money than they do, and Mark is happy to oblige. Mark also indicated that although he spends time with his friends, they are not close and does not feel like he has a close and supportive male friend.

Mark indicates that he also spends time with his business partner, Joe, although their friendship has waned in recent years. He states they have known each other for 12 years. Mark says he does not drink much while he is with Joe, since he is the only person who think sometimes Mark drinks too much. He also said Joe does not know about his most recent DWI arrest.

When asked whom Mark can call when the "crap hits the fan" in his life, he was at a loss. He claims to have friends, but nobody who he feels really knows him, his thoughts, feelings, and desires. He claims to be members of no support groups or organizations that he feels offer support. "You know what they say … a person can be alone in a 100,000-person stadium … that's me, I guess." He immediately laughed that off, claiming he is strong and always in control of his life. "I'm good. …"

Issues to Consider (Complete Based on Data Presented Above):

Strengths to Consider (Complete Based on Data Presented Above):

Motivation for Change (Each Treatable Problem; Include Justification):

Diagnoses (*DSM-5* diagnoses; Substance Use and Mental Health):

NARRATIVE ASSESSMENT

Treatment Plan
Client: Mark Johnson   Date:
Social Worker:

Treatment Recommendation
Modality:
Program name:
Type and frequency of counseling:

Other supportive services and activities:

Rationale for treatment recommendation:

Goals
Goal #1-
Objectives:

   A.
   B.

Goal #2-
Objectives:

   A.
   B.
   C.

Goal #3-
Objectives:

   A.
   B.
   C.
   D.

Goal #4-
Objectives:

    A.
    B.
    C.
    D.

Rationale for plan:

High-Risk Aftercare and Intervention Plan
Identified high-risk situations:

Developed strategies to cope with high-risk situations:

Social support:

24-hour crisis/safety plan:

REFERENCE

Johnson, J. L. (2004). *Fundamentals of substance abuse practice*. Wadsworth/Brooks Cole.

CHAPTER 6

Meet James Snyder

The Wonder Boy with Secrets

Jerry L. Johnson

INTRODUCTION

Meet James Snyder, a 26-year-old self-described "Wonder Boy." As is true for many people, how a person appears in public and how they lead their lives can differ greatly. In this case, James Snyder is a young man with a beautiful wife and two young children. He is a successful contractor with loving parents and siblings and who appears to have it all.

After reading James's revealing personal information acquired during his three-session assessment, you will learn how appearances can be deceiving. James may be young and successful today, but his Wonder Boy successful-builder image is not sitting on a solid and level foundation. As in other cases, experienced clinical practitioners rarely allow appearances and images to cloud their clinical perspective. They use their client engagement skills to allow them to gather deep client life information to paint a complete and multiple systemic picture of each client's life, to gain a picture of how somebody manages their daily life.

Beginning with a childhood with parents too consumed with their own problems to attend to their children, James has learned to manage in an "everybody-for-themselves" family and world. In doing so, he has led his life, with troubles brewing from an early age, by keeping himself and his family outside the gaze of their community, parents, friends, and associates. He even keeps himself and his troubles from his wife and kids. Hence, his Wonder Boy image can live on, without anyone noticing the contradictions. However, as is often the case, because his foundation is not strong, suddenly cracks began appearing in his image, leading him to my office for an assessment and hopefully some help.

As in the previous chapter, James Snyder's case is presented differently from the cases in the first three chapters. In those cases, authors took readers inside the actual sessions to hear some of the dialogue and understand the process of data collection and motivation, to allow readers to read what the experienced practitioners were thinking and planning as the sessions proceeded. It's almost as if our authors/practitioners were thinking out loud during their cases.

In this chapter, instead of being inside the sessions, we present a completed Client Assessment form, which includes the personal information and data collected during the assessment process. Following assessment protocol, each completed section of this assessment form contains data along with relevant personal quotes from the client. However, the sections are devoid of "clinical assessment thinking." That is, we have omitted the practitioner's thinking, conclusions, diagnostics, final assessment report, and treatment plan.

It is for the readers to read the case assessment report and complete each section based on the information contained in the client data. At the end of each section of the assessment form, there is space to write concluding paragraphs called "Issues to Consider" and "Strengths to Consider." Readers should complete these sections under each assessment dimension before moving to the end of chapter tasks.

After completing the Issues and Strengths sections throughout the chapter, at the end of the case, there are five important areas to be completed either alone, in groups, or as a class. These sections include:

1. **Clinical Diagnoses:** Readers will use the client information to make clinical diagnoses. There will be at least one substance use disorder and at least one mental health disorder. There may, in fact, be more.
2. **Stages of Change:** Readers will determine the relevant stage of change for each clinical diagnosis, along with the justification for said change (see Chapter 1 for more on the Stages of Change).
3. **Narrative Assessment:** Readers will write a complete narrative assessment, encompassing all client data, including clinical hypotheses and conclusions. This narrative must be holistic and be consistent with the clinical diagnoses made earlier (Johnson, 2004).
4. **Treatment Plan:** Using the information from above in combination with knowledge of treatment modalities, intensities, and methods, develop a treatment plan for James moving forward. The treatment plan will include treatment goals, measurable objectives, and a rationale for each section.
5. **High-Risk Aftercare and Intervention Plan:** Based on James's presentation and life circumstances, here you decide how his case will be handled in the event of any high-risk activities and behaviors and how these will be handled by the professionals and through recommendations or referrals for the client.

It is important to remember that all assessment and clinical conclusions, diagnoses, and decision making must be based on data contained in the case. That is, while it may be appropriate to speculate about issues based on new information learned later in therapy, any documented conclusions must have data to back them up. Conclusions without data represent the practitioner's implicit or explicit bias, out-of-control subjectivity, too much reliance on personal life experience, or simply overconfidence (Johnson, 2004).

Please take steps to help avoid making clinical decisions based on practitioner life experience, beliefs, attitudes, and thoughts. This exercise is good practice about an issue that professionals must be aware of throughout their clinical careers.

SUBSTANCE USE AND MENTAL HEALTH ASSESSMENT

Client name: James Snyder   Date of first contact: 0/0/00

Clinician: Date completed: 0/0/00

Client description, presenting problem, and context of referral

A. Brief Description of Client

James (Jim) is a 26-year-old White male, dressed casually and neatly, with the appearance of a healthy and successful person. He appeared well groomed, maintained appropriate eye contact, and offered a firm, professional handshake along with a look into my eyes. Once we began, Jim appeared polite but anxious during the sessions, at times perspiring and glancing quickly around the room. He also moved, tapped his feet, and seemed to have trouble sitting still during the sessions. He made good eye contact. He spoke rapidly and at length, often interrupting himself to make a different point. Jim appeared alone for this assessment. His spouse was invited but did not attend. Jim said they could not find child care. Jim said he has a wife of five years and two young daughters (two and four years old).

B. Chief Complaint and Symptoms by Client and Others

Jim's original complaint is that his "life is out of control," and he might need help "getting his act together." He said, "I'm known as the Wonder Boy around town, but I don't feel so wonderful these days." He got his nickname supposedly because he had become so successful in business at a young age, has a beautiful family, and apparently "a perfect life."

Jim complained that his wife and parents insist his drug use (cocaine) and alcohol use is the reason he "seems to be losing it." Jim strongly denied his cocaine and alcohol use was involved in his problems at this time. He believes the real reason is because he has always been a "nervous sort" and that lately (in the last six months) his nerves have "gotten worse." He claims to have trouble sleeping and his appetite is "weak." He claims to sleep on average two to three hours per night, but not "good sleep." Jim says he is "wide awake" at odd times and feels compelled to think about work, his family, and his hobby of building furniture. Jim claims he has fallen into the habit of building furniture late at night into the early morning when he cannot sleep. Recently, this has occurred more nights than not.

He also claims to have experienced "serious" periods of sadness at times in his life, especially during his teen years. "I'm not depressed like my mom, but I sure do get sad sometimes." During these periods, he is tired and lacks energy, but still cannot sleep or eat. He says he feels like the "weight of the world" is on his shoulders. He claims to have never told anybody, including his wife and parents, about this or his nervousness, as he does not want people to think he is "mentally ill."

Jim said that if his spouse or parents were in the session, they would blame his nerves, sadness, and other behavior on his cocaine and alcohol use. He does not think they believe he has legitimate mood problems (he has not told them). He said friends and coworkers would never know he has problems; they would say he was "high-strung" and full of energy, creative, and is driven. Jim said he wants therapy to help him learn to "relax and enjoy life again." He reiterated he did not believe his "occasional" use of cocaine and alcohol "to relax" is a problem.

C. Context of the Referral, Precipitating Events, Facts, and Dates

Jim says he "chose" to come in for an assessment and "therapy" on his own; that he was tired of feeling bad; and to prove to his wife and parents he does not have an alcohol and/or cocaine problem. He claims his decision to attend was not made under any outside pressure, yet he pointed out that there is a discrepancy between what he believes are his problems and what his spouse and family believe are the problems, and this has led to several loud and angry arguments. He also said his spouse "encouraged" him to come for therapy, but he did not feel as if he was being forced into it.

When asked about his reasons for coming now as opposed to a month ago, Jim said he chose to come for therapy today after experiencing "four straight sleepless nights and several arguments with his spouse" over his drug use and emerging family financial troubles. He claims that the "tension" in his life makes his moods swing from nervousness to sadness, and this is the reason for his sleepless nights and not cocaine use. He also claimed his "financial issues" are not related to any spending on cocaine, but on his wife's spending on "clothes and shoes."

Issues to Consider (Based on Data Recorded Above):

Strengths to Consider (Based on Data Recorded Above):

Substance Use and/or Mental Health Treatment History

A. Substance Abuse Treatment (Self and Family Members)
Jim said he has been using alcohol and drugs since he was 12 years old. He was a client in long-term residential substance abuse treatment program for his alcohol and marijuana use at 16 years old, resulting from problems in school attendance and a history of status offenses as a juvenile (see legal history). His treatment lasted six months and was followed by a recommendation to attend AA meetings (which he refused) and outpatient family therapy (which he and his family also refused). He said rehab was "a waste of time," and he only stayed the full term to please his parents and "get the school off my ass." He claims he was experiencing his "mood problems" during this time but never told his rehab counselor and was never asked about it. Like his parents and wife, Jim assumed the rehab counselor attributed his moods to "withdrawal" and being unable to "use," so he never asked about it.

B. Client Attitude Toward Treatment
When asked, Jim stated the treatment center experience was a "joke." He believed he had "no business" in a residential treatment program, given that his drug use was "minimal" at the time ("I'd only been drinking and smoking for four years by then"). He says his peers in the program were "far worse" than him, and he had "nothing in common" with any of them. He said that the program insisted he admit to having a "disease" (addiction) and be "powerless" over his use, and that he refused for a time. Jim said he finally admitted to having the "disease" because it was the only way he was ever going to complete the program and go home. Jim said "there is no way in hell" he believed his use was addiction then, or now, for that matter. He said he liked one of the counselors, but most of them were "lame-ass former drug addicts" who thought everyone who used alcohol and drugs was an addict.

Jim reported that his father was an inpatient alcohol treatment client several years ago for alcoholism and that he had been sober since that time (five years). His father is a current Alcoholics Anonymous (AA) member, and his mother and wife attend Al-Anon two to three times per week. He also stated that his paternal grandfather probably could have used treatment for alcoholism but never attended and died a "drunk." Jim thinks his wife and parents believe he has a serious substance use problem because they spend all their time in those "damned" meetings. "I think they want me to fit the profile of what they hear in AA and Al-Anon ... those people think everybody is an addict."

C. Mental Health Treatment

Jim reports no history of professional treatment for mental health problems. He says he had not told anyone, parents, wife, or his counselors in rehab about his "mood problems" discussed above and in more depth below under Mental Health Status. He does not think he is mentally ill, so he does not want to be sent to a "psychiatrist" to be certified "crazy." He claims to have never discussed his mood problems, as he calls them, with anybody until this session. He claims he decided to discuss them now because having mood problems is "probably" better than people thinking he's an addict.

His mother was on "some kind of medication" for depression for many years while his father was drinking. He says he believes she still takes her medication today. There were no reports of other family members attending mental health treatment.

D. Attitudes About Mental Health Treatment(s)

Jim said his mother's experience with medication for depression was excellent "for her, but it's not for me." It helped her "feel much better" and allowed her to function during a hard time in her parents' life. Jim has no experience to report on, although he does state he believes any talk of mental health issues means he is either "mentally ill" or "crazy."

Jim says his general attitude about counseling and therapy is "not good." "No offense, but I'm not sure you people ever help anybody."

Issues to Consider (Based on Data Recorded Above):

Strengths to Consider (Based on Data Above):

Substance Use History

A. Lifetime Substance Use History (Complete table. Explain in narrative.):

SUBSTANCE	FREQUENCY	DOSE (AVG.)	AGE AT FIRST USE	AGE AT LAST USE	ROUTE OF ADMIN.	OVER-DOSE
Alcohol (beer)	Daily	3–6 cans	12	N/A	Drink	No
Alcohol (liquor)	2–3 x's/week	2–3 shots/use	12	N/A	Drink	No
Cocaine (powder)	3–4 x's/week	¼ oz/week	23	N/A	Snort/smoke	No
Marijuana	1–2 x's/week	1 joint	12	N/A	Smoke	No
LSD	1 x/week	1 tab	14	18	Oral	Yes
"Speed"	2–3 x's/week	1–2 pills	14	23	Oral	No
Nicotine	Daily	1 can per day	19	N/A	Chewing	No

B. **Drugs used in previous 30 days:** Jim reported drinking and snorting cocaine the day before this session (his second). He also chews tobacco daily. In the 48 hours prior to the session, Jim claims he consumed at least 12 cans of beer and snorted at least 3 grams of powder cocaine, along with nicotine. Over the previous 30 days, it appears Jim drinks at least three to six beers and at least one shot of liquor on most days and smokes marijuana three to four times per week. He also snorts cocaine "3–4" times per week, anywhere from "one line" to a gram per use.

C. **Top three drugs of choice:** Jim claims cocaine, alcohol, and LSD as his current drugs of choice, although he quit using LSD when he was 18 years old after a "bad trip." He says his "acid days" were the most fun he ever had partying. He enjoyed being "lost" in a fantasy world. He says he would do LSD again if he weren't fearful of another bad trip.

He began using cocaine at age 23, and says cocaine makes him feel confident, strong, and smart and he really "loves" it. He began drinking and smoking marijuana at age 12 and has used both/and daily since that time, except when he was in rehab. He claims alcohol "makes me loose and takes the edge off," while marijuana helps him "chill and makes my appetite come back." His use history shows that Jim used what he called "speed" (amphetamines, diet pills, etc.; he did not say) from an early age until he apparently began using cocaine. This is noteworthy, since both drugs are stimulants.

D. **Drug mixing:** Jim constantly mixes three drugs: cocaine, alcohol, and nicotine. This mixture presents no clear and present health danger from an accidental overdose perspective. There is no evidence that Jim mixes any other depressant drugs with alcohol, as he reports that he does not take prescription medication and appears to favor stimulant drugs over depressant drugs.

E. **Longest period of abstinence:** Jim reports that he has not gone 24 hours without drinking or using drugs in the last 10 years. Until age 23, Jim primarily used either alcohol, marijuana, and speed daily since age 16. He says he began using cocaine and abandoned "speed" around age 23, three years earlier.

Jim states he is not worried by his daily use of multiple substances, since he only uses "casually" and is always able to cut down or quit if it was needed. He claims he has gone hours without using anything at all and has gone days without using some of his favorites, proving he doesn't "need" it. He claims his "youth" makes his use fine: "I'm not an old, weak fart … I'm strong!"

F. **Narrative (include attitudes and beliefs about use):** Jim began using alcohol, marijuana, and stimulant drugs at 12 years old and has been using on a regular daily basis since he was 16 (10 years). He began drinking and smoking with friends in school and began increasing his use as he moved into high school. He said his parents never said anything in the early years "because of Dad's drinking, they had their own problems." Jim began using cocaine (both snorting and smoking) since age 23, after using what he calls "speed" since he was 12.

His use is regular and consistent; he stated he has not been abstinent for more than 24 hours since he was 16, just out of substance abuse rehab. Jim has used alcohol and other drugs regularly, beginning at a young age. Moreover, he has used a mixture of drugs since that time. Based on his substance use history, while he has not used a plethora of drugs, it appears Jim finds certain drugs and mixtures that he likes and stays with them. He stopped using LSD, a drug he used weekly for five years, only after experiencing a "bad trip." This experience has made Jim afraid of LSD, despite his liking of the drug.

Another interesting point is his use of "speed" (amphetamines and other stimulants) until age 23, when he began using cocaine. Jim says he likes the stimulants better than other drugs. He reports that "90%" of his cocaine use is powder cocaine, but occasionally he will smoke crack cocaine for a new experience, and he especially likes the "rush" and the "explosion in my head" when he smokes crack cocaine. He admitted the amount of cocaine used each week has increased in the last year and even more in recent weeks. He also said he does not feel as good as he once did when using cocaine. He denied that his financial issues have anything to do with his increasing cocaine use, but rather were caused by his wife's spending habits.

Jim states that he has "no problem" with his substance use, and he is unashamed of it, even though his wife and parents are against it and believe it is a significant problem in his life. While he knows how destructive alcohol can be because of his father, Jim claims he is not a "drunk" who "needs it" every day. When asked about his daily use, Jim claimed he drinks to relax and have fun but does not "need it" to survive. When asked if he thought he had a drug problem, Jim stated, "No, I don't have a problem." However, he did say that he had thought about it before deciding that he "didn't need it, so I couldn't have a problem."

Jim reports being sent to residential substance abuse treatment for six months as an adolescent. He claims he did not need it, did not use enough to go to rehab, and had nothing in common with his peers. He refused aftercare AA meeting attendance, and his family never followed through with requested family therapy upon his release. He claims that rehab is "useless" for somebody like him because he does not have any problems with his use, and he certainly is "not an addict."

Jim also reports he has experienced a lifetime of "nervousness" and periods of "sadness" in his life. He claims he is "just high-strung," while his wife and parents believe these are side effects of his extensive drug use (see Mental Health Status). He claims that his use and the disagreement with his wife over it does not put his marriage at risk, but it does cause problems that must be fixed.

Issues to Consider (Based on Data Recorded Above):

Strengths to Consider (Based on Data Recorded Above):

Medical History

Jim reports no recurrent medical issues or problems, including any substance use problems. He has never had surgery or been hospitalized for any medical issues to this point in his life. As stated earlier, Jim was placed in a six-month adolescent substance abuse residential program at age 16.

Jim claims he attends "regular" physical examinations with his family doctor. He claims he is "young and strong" and has no health worries. He has not subjected himself to any drug testing or liver/kidney testing as part of his physical examinations, claiming he does not need to since he is "perfectly healthy."

Issues to Consider (Based on Data Recorded Above):

Strengths to Consider (Based on Data Recorded Above):

Basic Needs

Jim lives in his home (which he owns) with his wife and two children. He appears to be meeting his personal and family's basic needs. He is employed as a contractor, specializing in home building. He owns his own business and claims to "be busy" and "making great money." He claims that his family meets their food, clothing, shelter, and safety needs. He says the family is presently experiencing financial troubles, forcing him to expand his business and the number of jobs he takes on. He says that his wife blames his expensive cocaine use, but Jim blames the problems (while temporary) on his wife's out-of-control spending on "clothes and shoes."

He stated that he is the "wonder boy" in that he is a successful builder, bringing home more than $100,000 annually. When asked, Jim admitted to working when high on cocaine and that sometimes it made him a better builder because it "relaxes" him. He says his substance use causes no work problems "to speak of." He graduated from high school on time and said he never had the desire to go to college.

Issues to Consider (Based on Data Recorded Above):

Strengths to Consider (Based on Data Recorded Above):

Mental Health Status
Mental Status Screening (Check All That Apply):

A. **General appearance:**

1. Physical appearance: _X_ neat _X_ clean __unkempt __older __younger
X appropriate

2. Attitude:

_X_cooperative ___negative ___suspicious ___inaccessible ___shy ___frank

___hostile ___sensitive ___uncooperative ___quiet _X_ polite ___provocative

___resentful ___irritable ___submissive ___indifferent _X_ serious

_X_defensive _X_tense ___preoccupied ___detached

Explain: Jim presented with a clean and appropriate appearance and on time for his first appointment. He presented as cooperative, claiming that attending therapy was his idea. However, as the discussion moved into his personal substance use behaviors, Jim became tense and defensive, bordering on uncooperative. He began deflecting and blaming, mostly his wife and parents for misreading his substance use as a problem. He flatly denies having any issues or problems with his daily use of substances.

B. **Behavioral functioning:**

1. Motor activity:

___normal ___slow ___hyperactive

_X_ restless ___tremors _X_ agitation

___other: _____

2. Gait: _X_ normal ___stooped ___awkward ___staggering

3. Posture: _X_ normal ___rigid ___limp ___gesturing

Explain: Jim appeared to have trouble relaxing and sitting still. He made eye contact but also looked quickly around the room, was unsettled physically, tapping his feet and twisting his fingers. This could be a sign of being nervous in the first session but could also represent other issues. His activity did match his description of being "high-strung" and/or "nervous."

    C.   **Speech:**

___normal   _X_ spontaneous   ___slow   ___hesitant   _X_ rapid

___stutter   ___pressured   ___soft   _X_ loud   ___slurred

___monotonous   _X_ emotional   ___mumbled   ___threatening

Explain: Jim spoke rapidly, rushed, and without pause. His emotionality in his speech (sad, angry, defensive, defiant) was noteworthy. He was loud at times, so much so that people in the waiting room could hear, and at other times he spoke so softly he had to be asked to repeat himself. He laughed hard and loud, almost "deliriously" loud.

    D.   **Emotional Functioning:**

    1. Mood: _X_ euphoric   _X_ depressed   _X_ anxious   _X_ angry

    2. Affect:

        ___ appropriate   _X_ inappropriate   ___flat   _X_ broad

        ___constricted   ___blunted   _X_ euphoric

Explain: Jim's moods fluctuated from happy/euphoric, depressed, to angry and anxious. His mood was difficult to predict in that he would answer some difficult questions almost euphorically and some "easier" questions anxiously or angrily. His moods bounced and represented the spectrum during his sessions. Similarly, Jim's affect was both happy and unhappy, not often consistent with the tone and tenor of the session discussion.

    E.   **Thought process:**

      _X_ appropriate   ___blocking   ___preservation

      ___incoherent   ___circumstantiality   ___flight of ideas

      ___loose association   _X_ distractible

Explain: In concert with the inconsistencies noted above, Jim's thought processes bounced from periods of appropriateness to distractible, changing subjects, words, and ideas in mid-sentence.

F. **Thought content:**

    _X_ appropriate   ___obsessions   ___compulsions   ___preoccupied

    ___guilt   ___suicidal   ___homicidal   ___somatic concerns

    ___ideas of reference/influence   ___thought control   ___thought broadcasting   ___paranoia

Explain: There is no evidence of thought disorders or issues to note.

G. **Perceptions:**

1. Hallucinations: ___auditory   ___visual   ___tactile   _X_ none

Explain: No indication of perceptual issues or disorders.

B. **Cognitive functions:**

1. Consciousness: _X_ alert   ___confused   ___clouded   ___stuporous   ___apathetic

2. Orientation: _X_ normal   ___defective (time, place, person)

3. Memory: _X_ normal   ___defective (___remote ___recent ___now)

4. Attention/concentration: ___normal   _X_ impaired

Explain: Jim was alert, almost too much so, oriented X 3 with normal memory. Given all the data described above, his ability to concentrate and be consistently attentive demonstrated a level of impairment during the meetings. What is not known if this impairment was caused by nerves in therapy, substance use, mental health issues, or a combination thereof.

I. **Insight:** ___good   ___fair   _X_ poor

Explain: Jim demonstrated little capacity for insight into his life and circumstances during the interviews. He was able to discuss problems and behaviors that could be viewed as potentially problematic but was unable or unwilling to consider them to be problems in his life needing attention, instead blaming others for their ideas, and rationalizing his issues/symptoms as normal for his age.

J. **Judgment:** ___good   fair   _X_ poor

Explain: For many of the reasons listed above, Jim's judgment appears poor, especially his apparent dismissal of any potential health of life issues caused by long-term, heavy substance use and his reported lifetime history of mood issues. Jim presented as someone whose judgment at any given moment will be such to verify his beliefs, desires, and needs above others.

Mental Status Impressions (Potential Mood, Anxiety, Thought, or Personality Disorders)

Jim presented with a clean and appropriate appearance and on time for his first appointment. He was mostly cooperative, claiming that attending therapy was his idea because his "life was out of control." However, as the discussion moved into his personal behaviors and moods, Jim became tense and defensive, sometimes bordering on uncooperative. He was able to freely discuss his symptoms but strongly resisted any suggestions these symptoms represented "problems" of any note. At this suggestion, Jim would deflect and blame others, mostly his wife and parents for talking about them or telling others because he would be labeled. He flatly denies having any mental health issues or problems that need treatment.

Jim appeared to have trouble sitting still, with nervous body energy throughout. He made eye contact occasionally but also looked quickly around the room, was unsettled physically, tapping his feet and twisting his fingers. This could be a sign of being nervous in his first session but could also represent other issues. His activity did match his description of being "high-strung" and/or "nervous."

Jim spoke rapidly, rushed, and without pause. His emotionality in his speech (sad, angry, defensive, defiant) was noteworthy and inconsistent. He was loud at times, so much so that people in the waiting room could hear, and at other times he spoke so softly he had to be asked to repeat himself. He laughed hard and loud, almost "deliriously" loud. His emotionality was often mismatched to the content of the discussion, making his emotional reactions difficult to predict and understand.

Jim's moods fluctuated from happy/euphoric, depressed, to angry and anxious. His mood was difficult to predict in that he would answer some difficult questions almost euphorically and some "easier" questions anxiously or angrily. His moods bounced and represented the spectrum during his sessions. Similarly, Jim's affect was both happy and unhappy, not often consistent with the tone and tenor of the session discussion. He was often anxious, moving between being agitated and restless to being listless and resigned.

He described a lifetime of being nervous and "high-strung." He described times where he exhibited high energy for days at a time, causing him to get little sleep and not eat. During these periods, Jim would stay up nights building furniture in his home shop and then work all day without needing sleep. Jim said he enjoyed these periods and enjoyed being so "full of energy." Often, these periods would be followed by shorter periods of sadness and being tired, restless, and irritable. He still reported difficulty sleeping during these periods. His nervousness began in his childhood but intensified as he became an older adolescent. He also said he was able to manage himself with his alcohol and drug use, as these seemed to enhance the moods he likes and moderate the moods he dislikes.

Jim reported no evidence of thought disorders or issues to note, and there were no indications of perceptual issues or disorders.

Jim was alert, almost too much so, oriented X 3 with normal memory. Given all the data described above, his ability to concentrate and be consistently attentive demonstrated a level of impairment during the meetings. What is not known if this impairment was caused by nerves in therapy, substance use, mental health issues, or a combination thereof.

Jim denies any thoughts of suicide or homicide, now or in the past.

Jim demonstrated little capacity for insight into his life and circumstances during the interviews. He was able to discuss problems and behaviors that could be viewed as potentially problematic but was unable or unwilling to consider them to be problems in his life needing attention, instead blaming others for their ideas and rationalizing his issues/symptoms as normal for his age.

For many of the reasons listed above, Jim's judgment appears poor, especially his apparent dismissal of any potential health of life issues caused by long-term, heavy substance use and his reported lifetime history of mood issues. Jim presented as someone whose judgment at any given moment will be such to verify his beliefs, desires, and needs above others.

Issues to Consider (Based on Data Reported Above):

Strengths to Consider (Based on Data Reported Above):

Family History and Structure

Jim is the eldest son of his parents, both of whom are living. He has two younger sisters: one is 23 years old and in college, and the other is 18 years old and living at home. His father is a recovering alcoholic who has been an AA member for five years, and his mother attends Al-Anon. Jim claims that he is currently close with his family members, although relations have been strained lately because of his father's insistence that he has a drug problem. Jim reports that his father drank heavily for most of his life, making him and his mother inaccessible because of their problems. He claims he had to raise and manage himself as a child because his parents were "overwhelmed." Jim states his sisters do not use or abuse alcohol and other drugs.

There is no evidence of physical, sexual, or emotional abuse in Jim's family, past or present. He says his father was not a "mean drunk" but was always out with friends drinking at bars and pubs. His mother and father rarely argued in front of the kids. According to Jim, it was hard to even know there were problems if one did not already know. His family, according to Jim, did not talk or communicate about problems and troubles, did not support each other emotionally, and everybody (including the kids) was left to "find their own way" and make their own decisions. Because of the troubles with his father's drinking and mother's depression dominating their lives, for the kids it was "everybody for themselves."

Jim's wife (Marie) is the only child of two living parents. She is a part-time secretary, working two days per week. According to Jim, there is no history of substance abuse or mental health problems in her family. Her family is close to his children and has expressed their belief that Jim has problems and needs help. Jim believes his mother-in-law has influenced Marie's opinion of his use over the last few months and blames his mother-in-law (and his parents) for some of the troubles between Marie and himself.

Jim and Marie have two young children: a boy (Jim Jr.) who is four years old and a girl (Ann-Marie) who is two. Jim and Marie have been married five years, and both pregnancies were planned. He reports that he "loves" his kids and wife and would not want to see anything happen to break up his family. He also says he is a good parent but works most of the time so he does not get to spend as much time with them as he would like.

His relationship with his wife has been strained lately over his substance use, financial problems, and recent evidence of sexual problems. According to Jim, over the last few months Marie has lost interest in sex, and at times, he is unable to perform. Jim claims that he has not had extramarital affairs and is loyal to his wife. He does not believe Marie is involved in extramarital relationships, either. When asked why Marie did not come to this session, Jim claims that they could not arrange child care. Jim agreed to bring Marie to a future session.

Jim says he does not believe his marriage is "in trouble," but they are just going through a difficult time. Jim does not believe these difficult times are related to him at all and that Marie just needs time to figure him out.

Jim's grandparents are all deceased. However, he claims that his paternal grandfather had drinking problems that contributed to his death.

Issues to Consider (Based on Data Reported Above):

Strengths to Consider (Based on Data Presented Above):

Social Support and Engagement

According to Jim, he has few friends and "nobody" he considers "close," except his wife. Jim says he has never been someone to have "lots" of friends or hang out in groups, instead preferring to have one or two "buddies" and "keep my own company."

He says his family was not one who had friends and family around. He does not remember attending social engagements as a child and rarely had friends over to play. As he grew older, he says he "just felt better" without a lot of people "knowing my business." He says he "hated" all the groups when he was in rehab and tried to keep to himself most of the time.

He states that he was once a good athlete and enjoyed golf after high school. However, he quit golfing three years ago and has not participated in sports of any kind since that time. He says that his goal, when not working, is to relax and "be calm" and that he is able to do that without needing people around. He enjoys working and building furniture in his shop. In fact, Jim states he cannot remember the last time his friends were together. When asked about this, he became agitated, saying, "There's nothing wrong not liking to be around people."

Jim states he has no social media involvement. He consistently said he does not like people to know too much about him, so he keeps to himself as much as possible. When asked whom he would call for support if his life fell apart, Jim said his wife, but he can handle whatever comes up, "like I have always done since I was a kid."

Jim and Marie live in a middle-class neighborhood that is a mixture of young and older families. They have lived in this home and neighborhood for three years. He claims his neighbors are friendly but distant, and that is "okay" with him. He has befriended one neighbor, with whom he likes to "party" on occasion. According to Jim, this person has become his sole source for cocaine. He finds the neighborhood safe and supportive of young families. Jim is largely disconnected and disengaged from neighbors, friends, and outside support.

Issues to Consider (Based on Data Reported Above):

Strengths to Consider (Based on Data Reported Above):

Legal History

As a juvenile, Jim was arrested at least five times for status offenses, including truancy, curfew violations, and two minor-in-possession-of-alcohol charges. As an adult, Jim had been arrested for drunk driving once two years earlier. He was given a suspended sentence, one year probation, and a restricted driver's license, all of which have ended. He claims the arrest was the most embarrassing moment of his life and vowed never to be arrested again. When asked, Jim admitted that he continues to drink and drive but that now he "knows how to get away with it."

Issues to Consider (Based on Data Reported Above):

Strengths to Consider (Based on Data Above):

Cultural Background and Engagement

Jim is a European American male of Italian descent, although he admits he has no connection to his Italian heritage. His wife is also Italian, and her family, according to Jim, does practice and abide by some of their Italian traditions, especially Catholicism. Jim attends church only to appease his wife and "to be a good role model" for his children. He believes the people in his church are "hypocrites" who act "pious" on Sunday, then return home and act differently. He denies any religious or spiritual beliefs, claiming he is a self-reliant man who does not need God or some other person telling him how to live his life. He identifies as a conservative Republican who is patriotic, loyal to and loves his country. He also said people should be more like him, able to take care of themselves and not need other people—"just do it, and don't whine."

Jim claims that he has never been one to "fit in" with groups, that he likes to be alone or with a small group of people. He claims that he fits best with the few friends with whom he can "relax" and "party" because they understand how tense he is and what his use does to make his life easier. Jim claims that his wife was once someone with whom he could relax, but that has changed recently. He claims that "nobody really knows me" and that he just wants to be left alone to live and "provide for his family." Jim's major daily goals are to "work, love his kids, and relax." According to Jim, the only way that he has "ever" found to relax is through substance use.

Issues to Consider (Based on Data Reported Above):

Strengths to Consider (Based on Data Reported Above):

Clinical Diagnoses (Substance Use and/or Mental Health with Rationale):

Justification:

Client Motivation (Stage of Change and Justification for Each Diagnosable Problem):

Issues to Consider (Based on Data Reported Above):

Strengths to Consider (Based on Data Reported Above):

Narrative Assessment (Include All Relevant Issues and Strengths to Compose a Multi-Systemic Description of the Client's Life):

Treatment Plan
Client: James Snyder   Date:
Social Worker:

Treatment Recommendation

    A. Modality:
    B. Program name:
    C. Type and frequency of counseling:

    D. Other supportive services and activities:

Rationale for treatment recommendation:

Goals
Goal #1-
Objectives:

    A.
    B.

Goal #2-
Objectives:

    A.
    B.
    C.

Goal #3-
Objectives:

    A.
    B.
    C.
    D.

Goal #4-
Objectives:

    A.
    B.
    C.
    D.

Rationale for plan:

High-Risk Aftercare and Intervention Plan
Identified high-risk situations:

Developed strategies to cope with high-risk situations:

Social support:

24-hour crisis/safety plan:

REFERENCE

Johnson, J. L. (2004). *Fundamentals of substance abuse practice.* Wadsworth/Brooks Cole.

CHAPTER 7

Co-Occurring Disorders Treatment
Best Practices

Jerry L. Johnson and Glen Brookhouse

INTRODUCTION

In this chapter, we look at the latest evidence regarding treatment outcomes, for treatment models and approaches, and modalities (outpatient, residential, etc.) pertaining to persons with co-occurring disorders. This chapter also explores the idea of integrated treatment for people with co-occurring disorders. While the idea of integrated treatment makes sense and is seen as best practice, we discover that most clients with co-occurring disorders do not experience integrated treatment. Studies have demonstrated the likelihood of poorer outcomes for clients participating in programs that do not offer specialized, integrated care (Compton et al., 2000).

We also look at which treatment modalities prove most effective with clients experiencing co-occurring disorders. While there is limited information available in this area, the literature again points to the need for integrated treatment (for both mental health and substance use disorders) together, ensuring clients never approach the "wrong door" when seeking help (SAMHSA, 2005).

OVERVIEW

Since the 1970s, practitioners have recognized the existence of substance use and mental health disorders in large numbers on professional caseloads (Woody & Blaine, 1979). Originally called dual diagnosis and/or dual disorders, professionals soon realized the coexistence of these disorders in individual clients often had major implications for treatment.

In the 1980s and 1990s, both substance use and mental health professionals found a wide range of mental health disorders were associated with substance abuse (De Leon, 1989; Pepper et al., 1981; Rounsaville et al., 1982;

Sciacca, 1991). Studies conducted in substance abuse programs typically report that 50–75% of clients have some type of co-occurring mental health disorder. Studies of mental health caseloads reported from 25–60% had co-occurring substance use disorders (Johnson, 2004).

Researchers in mental health not only found a link between the disorders but also discovered the complicating presence substance use has on treatment outcomes for mental health disorders, and vice versa. One study of 121 clients with psychoses found that participants with co-occurring substance use disorders (36%) spent twice as many days in the hospital over the two years prior to treatment as did clients without substance use problems (Crome 1999; Menezes et al., 1996). In addition, these clients had poorer outcomes, higher rates of HIV infection, relapse, rehospitalization, depression, and suicide risk (Drake et al., 1998; Office of the Surgeon General, 1999).

The assessment and treatment of clients with co-occurring mental health and substance use disorders present unique challenges to practitioners compared to clients with either a mental health or substance use disorder alone. That is, not only do the symptoms of each disorder(s) interact to make assessment and diagnoses difficult at best, but the intensity of each issue also interacts to make treatment retention and success a challenge. The Substance Abuse and Mental Health Services Administration (SAMHSA) defines co-occurring disorders as the presence of at least one mental health disorder coexisting with at least one substance use disorder, as defined by the *Diagnostic and Statistical Manual*-5th edition (APA, 2018).

The first step is often the most difficult: to determine if, in fact, co-occurring mental health and substance use disorders exist. This is often difficult because the effects of many drugs mimic a mental health disorder and vice versa, making it hard to discriminate between mental health disorders, mental health disorders caused by substance use, and/or behaviors that appear to be mental health disorders but are simply the side effects of substance use.

Ideally, to accurately assess mental health disorders, practitioners need clients to experience a period of substance use abstinence of at least a month or more (Flynn & Brown, 2008); some say 90 days is the optimal time for the most accurate results (Johnson, 2004). This period of abstinence allows clinicians to avoid confusing the client presenting symptoms with the normal effects of substance use (SAMHSA, 2005; Hasin, Trautman, & Endicott, 1998; Quello, Brady, & Sonne, 2005).

However, organizations and funding sources do not allow for this length of deliberation before making diagnoses. Therefore, practitioners often must adapt to practice in less than ideal conditions, trying to account for the possibility of assessment and diagnoses that is incomplete at best and, at worst, inaccurate.

In this situation, practitioners often over-identify mental health disorders (Flynn & Brown, 2008; Johnson, 2004). Because of the high risk for error in early diagnosis, some suggest that practitioners should perform multiple assessments over time (SAMHSA, 2005) after providing a "rule-out" diagnosis for possible mental health disorders (Johnson, 2004). Others suggest waiting to assess mental health disorders, employing quick screening instruments to determine if a full assessment is necessary later (Quello et al., 2005).

TREATING CO-OCCURRING DISORDERS IN SINGLE-FOCUS SUBSTANCE ABUSE PROGRAMS

As we demonstrate, the jury is still out about the most effective ways to help clients with multiple disorders, beyond recognizing that a "one-size-fits-all" approach does not work (Johnson, 2004). Similarly, current beliefs suggest that neither the mental health nor substance abuse treatment systems can provide adequate treatment alone for both mental health and substance use disorders.

Yet, there is evidence-based reason to believe that traditional forms of substance abuse treatment effects positive change in mental health and behavioral problems as a usual part of its work. Research and evaluation have often discovered that traditional substance abuse treatment, without enhancements to account for mental health disorders, are able to modify the psychological functioning of substance abuse clients (Brook & Whitehead, 1980; De Leon, 1984; 1989).

De Leon and Jainchill (1982) reported positive change in ratings of depression, self-esteem, and other psychological factors through traditional therapeutic community (long-term residential) treatments. However, the extent to which these individuals demonstrated mental health disorders and the severity of the disorders was not discussed. Other studies have examined treatment outcomes for individuals identified as exhibiting co-occurring disorders and substance use only. Surprisingly, while mental health disorders are often believed to have a negative effect on outcomes (including in this text), findings suggest that, in several instances, equally positive treatment outcomes were found for adults with and without diagnosable mental health disorders and troubling behavioral symptoms (Nace & Davis, 1993; Ross, Dermatis, Levounis, & Galanter, 2003), and adolescents (Grella, Joshi, & Hser, 2003). Similarly, a study involving more than 1000 clients admitted to 39 programs representing all major modalities reported no differences in outcomes for individuals with co-occurring disorders treated with mental health services and those treated with traditional substance abuse treatment, including outcomes for measures of mental health symptom severity (Hser, Grella, Evans, & Huang, 2006).

Researchers also demonstrated that substance abuse treatment for clients with co-occurring mental health disorders can be beneficial—even for clients with serious mental health symptoms. For example, the National Treatment Improvement Evaluation Study (NTIES) found marked reductions in suicidality the year following substance abuse treatment compared to the year prior to treatment, for both males and females. Suicide attempts declined about four-fifths for both the 3,037 male clients and the 1,374 female clients studied (Karageorge, 2001). Many clients in traditional substance abuse treatment settings with mild-to-moderate mental health disorders were found to do well with traditional substance abuse treatment methods (Hser et al., 2001; Hubbard et al., 1989; Joe et al., 1995; Simpson et al., 2002; Woody et al., 1991).

These findings do nothing to limit the importance of providing effective treatment services, including mental health services, for the significant number of clients whose severity of disorder indicates the need for those services. What they suggest is that, in a time of diminished resources, all is not lost for clients with certain types of co-occurring disorders.

It is also important to remember that these studies did not discuss the severity of the substance use and/or mental health disorders. So, it is impossible to know, or suggest, that clients with moderate-to-severe mental health disorders would fare as well in substance abuse–only treatment programs. To this day, perhaps the greatest challenge remaining is for clients with more serious mental health disorders (SAMHSA, 2005).

According to Flynn and Brown (2008), an important issue in the field is that the term "co-occurring disorder" is a blanket descriptor covering all types of substance use and mental health disorders, including all levels of severity. Little has been done to distinguish between the severity of mental health disorders and substance use disorders. Watkins and colleagues (Watkins et al., 2005) point out that the variety of mental health disorders and substance use disorders make it difficult to gather efficacy data for all the potential combinations. They also suggest a research strategy based on either or both the prevalence and clinical significance of combinations. This is based on research showing that differences in treatment outcomes are associated with diagnostic differences (Compton et al., 2003).

CURRENT BEST PRACTICES

Integrated Care

Historically, clients with co-occurring disorders have been treated by multiple providers, each specializing in either substance use or mental health disorders, often at different agencies or locations. The pitfalls of this approach are many, including difficulty coordinating treatment planning and intervention. It also forces clients into multiple appointments in multiple locations, leading to higher dropout rates and a lack of coordinated progress (Flynn & Brown, 2008).

The conventional boundaries between single-focus agencies (i.e., either substance abuse or mental health) presents barriers to the progress of clients with co-occurring disorders (Baker, 1991). Therefore, treating clients effectively for co-occurring disorders represents a challenge to traditional treatment systems, to the limited resources often allocated for treatment, and to prevailing notions about professional education and training.

For example, even today, most professional graduate schools require students to specialize either by modality or field of practice (i.e., mental health, child welfare, substance use) while agencies adhere to a narrow focus regarding accepted client populations and/or fields of practice. Many social agencies and professional schools have not changed to accommodate clients with co-occurring disorders. Therefore, both the treatment and education systems encourage the type of focus that often leads to the inability to recognize or consider that a second (or third) disorder may in fact, exist. Moreover, graduating students entering the professions are unprepared for current co-occurring disorder treatments and approaches that require integrated care.

Beyond providing care that specifically addresses both categories of problem, the misinterpretation of co-occurring disorders and/or failure to identify a co-occurring mental health disorder is often a detriment to treatment. For example, the symptoms of a co-occurring mental health disorder are often misinterpreted by substance abuse professionals as poor or incomplete "recovery" from chemical dependency. Mental health specialists often fail to ask about substance use, assuming the symptoms they see—which may be caused by substance abuse—are evidence of diagnosable mental health symptoms. Mental health disorders interfere with a client's ability and motivation to participate in substance abuse treatment, and vice versa. Unfortunately, these clients are often labeled "resistant" and "not ready for treatment" by substance abuse and mental health professionals when they often have good reason for their behavior.

For example, individuals suffering from anxiety disorders may fear and/or resist attending support groups or group therapy sessions. Depressed clients may be too unmotivated and lethargic to participate in treatment. Those with psychotic or manic symptoms may exhibit bizarre behavior and poor personal relations in treatment. Clients whose substance use is the primary way of suppressing mental health symptoms (self-medication) may not progress toward, achieve, and/or maintain abstinence in the time or with the consistency that substance use professionals prefer (Denning, 2000).

There remain instances where substance abuse professionals consider clients with mental health disorders, taking prescribed medication to treat those disorders, as not being abstinent; in other words, in perpetual relapse. There are reports of substance abuse professionals demanding these clients stop using medications in order to find "recovery," and any use of prescribed medication is considered a relapse (Johnson, 2004). The bottom line is this: failure to identify co-occurring mental health symptoms often end with a client being removed or barred from treatment at a time when they are most vulnerable.

From a mental health practitioner perspective, failure to recognize and assess client's substance use history can be deadly. For example, many clients receiving mental health treatment take prescribed medications for their disorders. If a client's substance use is not detected and they continue using alcohol and/or other drugs in combination with prescribed medication, they are at risk of accidental overdose and even death. Moreover, as stated above, many of the desired side effects of substance use mimic mental health disorder symptoms, leading to misdiagnoses, mismatched treatment planning, and ineffective intervention plans that do not address the multifaceted nature of the client's problems (Johnson, 2004; Denning, 2000).

For example, stimulant drugs (methamphetamine, cocaine, etc.) taken in large amounts often lead to a psychosis that appears the same as someone having a legitimate psychotic episode. Without the knowledge of their substance use history and the skills to assess, diagnose, and treat these issues, this client may end up on inappropriate medications with a mismatched diagnosis and treatment regimen.

Given these issues, the idea of practicing integrated care based on the coordination of substance use and mental health services within a single site or between treatment sites has emerged in the last 20 years. As described by Mueser and colleagues (2003), integrated treatment is the seamless integration of mental health and substance abuse interventions in order to form a cohesive, unitary system of care. This means the best possible care, in theory, occurs when this seamless integration is available by providing mental health and substance use services simultaneously in the same agency and/or by the same clinicians.

Yet, there is little agreement on a working definition of integrated treatment (Watkins et al., 2005). Integrated treatment is defined both as services co-located in one site, requiring staff cross-trained in both disciplines and as a system of care involving services provided through referrals across organizations. Literature reviews over the years regarding the efficacy of integrated treatment show considerable support for its effectiveness for co-occurring disorders (Drake et al., 2004; Meuser et al., 2003). Others (Donald, Dower, & Kavanagh, 2005) conclude the findings from randomized clinical trials regarding the efficacy of integrated treatment remain inconclusive.

Drake and colleagues (cf. Mueser, Torrey, & Lynde, 2003) developed an integrated dual disorder treatment (IDDT) provided in community mental health settings for clients with severe mental illness and substance use disorders. Moreover, strategies for matching treatments to client symptom severity are now beginning to appear. Chen et al. (2006) demonstrated that high-severity clients matched to higher-intensity treatments had better psychiatric and substance use outcomes than those treated in low-intensity programs. They further report that "moderate-severity [dual diagnosis] patients" had positive and comparable treatment outcomes whether treated in high or low service-intensity programs, whereas "high-severity [dual diagnosis] patients" exposed to high service-intensity programs had better substance abuse and psychiatric outcomes than those exposed to low service-intensity programs. Similarly, Curran and colleagues (Curran, Kirchner, Worley, Rookey, & Booth, 2002) report that severity of depressive symptomatology, rather than the simple presence or absence of diagnosable depression, helped to predict program retention.

The extent to which clients entering both substance abuse and mental health treatment programs for co-occurring disorders, in combination with the expressed support for integrated treatment, even if it is less than uniform, appears to suggest that integrated treatment is widely implemented by treatment programs. Yet, research suggests that only 7–8% of clients with co-occurring disorders received both substance abuse and mental health services simultaneously (Harris & Edlund, 2005; Watkins et al., 2001), although 15% of clients with substance use disorders and serious mental disorder received integrated care (Harris & Edlund, 2005). If this evidence is true, it appears the profession has a long way to go before realizing the benefits of effectively cross-trained, co-occurring disorder integrated treatment programs.

However, as earlier findings suggest, perhaps substance abuse treatment should not be viewed as so single focused that achievement beyond the level of change in substance use and antisocial behaviors is either unlikely or limited. In the case where programs are not integrated and/or where clients lack access to integrated care, substance abuse professionals should follow the lead of their clients in terms of mental health problems and coping difficulties and work with clients to resolve these issues. Moreover, as clients find success in coping with problems in one area of living, they can begin feeling an increased sense of self and/or self-efficacy that improves the confidence to change behaviors in other areas of life. Individuals with less severe mental health problems may show improved psychological functioning related to reduced substance use in traditional substance abuse treatment programs (Flynn & Brown, 2008).

The Four Quadrants of Care

In the early 1990s, in conjunction with SAMHSA, Ries (1993) developed a conceptual framework to classify clients into four basic groups based on relative symptom severity, not diagnosis (SAMHSA, 2005). The four-quadrant model has two distinct uses:

1. To help conceptualize an individual client's treatment needs based on the assessed and demonstrated severity of their symptoms of both substance use and mental health issues.

2. In lieu of a fully integrated co-occurring disorders treatment system, the four-quadrant model helps practitioners understand where certain severities of co-occurring disorders can effectively find treatment.

The four Quadrants of Care include:

Quadrant I: Clients who fall into this quadrant include individuals with <u>low-severity substance use and low-severity mental health disorders</u>. These low-severity clients can often have their treatment needs met in normal outpatient settings in either substance use or mental health agencies, if both disorders are identified and treated, and the staff are trained in both.

Quadrant II: Clients in this quadrant include people with <u>high-severity mental health disorders</u> who are usually identified as priority clients within the mental health system. Quadrant II clients will also have <u>low-severity substance use disorders</u> (i.e., client in sobriety, or partial sobriety, and/or relapse). These clients are often best served in continuing care in the mental health system and will likely be well served in many intermediate-care mental health programs using case management. Again, this is based on cross-trained professional staff who identify both disorders.

Quadrant III: This quadrant includes clients with <u>high-severity substance use disorders and low-to-moderate-severity mental health disorders.</u> These clients are generally well served in intermediate substance abuse programs (i.e., intensive outpatient, short-term inpatient, detox centers followed by outpatient, etc.). Again, success for clients in this quadrant depends on the substance abuse professionals being well trained in mental health disorders, with access to the appropriate services that may be required (i.e., psychiatrist for medication management).

Quadrant IV: Because of its seriousness and intensity, this quadrant is subdivided into two subgroups.

- This subgroup includes individuals with <u>serious and persistent mental illness (SPMI) who also have severe and unstable substance use disorders.</u>
- The second subgroup includes individuals with <u>severe and unstable substance use disorders and high-severity behavioral problems (violent tendencies, high suicidality, etc.) who do not yet meet the criteria for SPMI.</u>

Individuals who meet the criteria for both subgroups require intensive, comprehensive, and integrated services for both their substance use and mental health disorders. Treatment is often located in intensive inpatient programs specializing in both, state hospitals, therapeutic communities, long-term residential programs, and/or a jail or prison program. Often, these clients come to the attention of the treatment community through emergency rooms and/or law enforcement (SAMHSA, 2005).

Any chances for treatment success using the four quadrants of care rely on effective staff training and experience in identifying and working with both mental health and substance use disorders. Practitioners are encouraged to locate consultants to advise if their training and experience are lacking in either substance use or mental health assessment and treatment.

Treatment Models and Methods: Current Findings

Current practice research is mixed on the best methods, models, and lengths of service for clients with co-occurring disorders. Several studies reported on more short-term effects, while few examined outcomes over a longer term (beyond two years). This is unfortunate, as there is some indication that co-occurring disorders treatment is most effective—in fact, only effective—in association with long-term treatments without time limits (Meuser, Torrey, & Lynde, 2003). Others also emphasized a longitudinal perspective when treating co-occurring disorders, specifically highlighting the importance of continuity of care involving an extended, multiyear period (Drake, Wallach, & McGovern, 2005; Osher, 1996). For example, of the materials reviewed for this chapter, several studies reported data with 12-month results (Baker et al., 2012; Bowen et al., 2014; Cornelius et al., 2011; Pennay et al., 2011; Riper et al., 2014). Few (Pennay et al., 2011) reported 16-month and/or longer follow-up (Cornelius et al., 2011).

It appears that Cognitive Behavioral Therapy (CBT) and Motivational Interviewing (MI) are the most frequently measured and reported methods by researchers. For example, one study measured the impact of CBT on PTSD (McGovern et al., 2009). The results showed that 27% of the participants at post-treatment remained "positive" for PTSD, while 20% were PTSD-positive at three-month follow-up. Researchers in this study stated that participants who received CBT for PTSD symptoms demonstrated significant reductions in substance use and in substance use severity (McGovern et al., 2009). Using an estimate of client retention (those who attended 75% of scheduled sessions) as its threshold, researchers reported that 65% of original patients completed the course of therapy (McGovern et al., 2009). However, although the retention rate compares favorably to other treatments for co-occurring PTSD and substance use, treatment engagement and completion remains a challenge for these patients.

Similarly, another study regarding clients with co-occurring PTSD and substance use disorders found that participants with severe PTSD assigned to more traditional individual addiction counseling were less likely to participate than participants assigned to individual addiction counseling using an integrated CBT approach (McGovern et al., 2011). Further, the study showed a significant reduction in PTSD symptoms when CBT was integrated with individual addiction therapy. A meaningful reduction in PTSD symptoms, according to the CAPS-PTSD (used in this study) scale, is 15 points or more (Weathers, Ruscio, & Keane, 1999).

McGovern et al. (2011) reported an average 40-point reduction from baseline to post-treatment and an average of 30-point reduction at three-month follow-up.

The same study compared the impact of more traditional individual addiction counseling (non-CBT and community support groups) and CBT-based individual addiction counseling. McGovern et al. (2011) found that both treatment conditions were similarly effective in reducing substance use. Others have found that positive changes in PTSD symptoms were a precursor to later changes in substance use behaviors (McGovern et al., 2011; Back et al., 2006; Hien et al., 2010). Moreover, CBT was also found to reduce both substance use and depression symptoms (Brown, Evans, Miller, Burgess, & Mueller, 1997) and substance use and PTSD symptoms (Hien, Cohen, Miele, Litt, & Capstick, 2004).

Other research examined the integration of CBT with outpatient treatment for depressive symptoms and substance use (Hunter et al., 2012). This research found that CBT integration in treatment "holds promise" for treating both depressive symptoms and substance use (Hunter et al., 2012). Hunter and colleagues (2012) claimed that the range of confidence intervals in the study suggests that CBT integration with traditional outpatient care is likely to lead to reductions in symptoms as compared to "usual" care, although the study reported no actual reductions when compared to traditional substance use outpatient treatment (Hunter et al., 2012).

Similarly, Riper et al. (2014) conducted a meta-analysis to review the impact of CBT and Motivational Interviewing (MI) of co-occurring alcohol use disorders and depression. The researchers found this combination caused a small but significant reduction in alcohol use, with the results similar for depression (Riper et al., 2014). At 12-month follow-up, researchers performed comprehensive client assessment that demonstrated the small but significant changes in depression symptoms were maintained, but with a trend toward significance. There was no report of whether positive changes reported in alcohol use were maintained at the 12-month follow-up (Riper et al., 2014).

In a systematic review about the efficacy of Motivational Interviewing and CBT treatments based on seven controlled studies (Baker et al., 2012), researchers concluded:

1. Brief interventions, based on MI, appear effective and may achieve a reduction in alcohol consumption for many people.
2. Longer courses of CBT (e.g., 10 sessions) treatment appear to be associated with improvements in mental health–related domains of functioning.

Baker et al. (2012) concluded that people with co-occurring disorders should be initially offered low-intensity, brief MI interventions for their substance use disorders. This can be followed by more intensive CBT interventions to treat existing mental health disorders if needed. The researchers did not include any information about the severity of the disorders. That is, based on this review, it is unknown whether these recommendations are effective with different problem severities or only low-severity disorders.

Hides et al. (2011) examined the effect CBT and MI treatments had on young adults (16–25) when these methods were added to standard care (SC) practices (SC+CBT/MI). The researchers examined clients with diagnosed mood disorders, anxiety disorders, and comorbid anxiety and mood disorder, coexisting with cannabis, alcohol, and opiate use.

Researchers reported the reduction in cannabis use was significantly greater than the use of other substances from baseline to three months in the SC+CBT/MI group compared to clients in standard care (Hides et al., 2011). They also claimed that these clients were less likely to be in the precontemplation stage of change after three months in the program. The study also found a significant reduction in depression scores from baseline to three and six months. Youth in the standard care group also reported reduced depression scores at six months, but not between baseline and three months (Hides et al., 2011).

Delivery of SC+CBT/MI was associated with treatment progress with respect to depression, substance use, motivation to change, and frequency of social contacts in the first three months. According to Hides et al. (2011), these results provide some indication of a change in vulnerability factors, thought to underlie depression and substance use as a result of enhanced care. Yet, researchers also found that all participants, regardless of treatment group, reported improved functionality and quality of life after six months of treatment (Hides et al., 2011).

A different study looked at the effects of Motivational Enhancement Therapy (MET) and CBT on Major Depressive Disorder co-occurring with an Alcohol Use Disorder in adolescents (Cornelius et al., 2011). Clients participated in a structured program that used a preplanned manual with CBT/MET tenets during the acute treatment phase. Researchers claim these clients demonstrated greater improvements in symptoms of depression and alcohol use at the two-year follow-up compared to clients receiving more traditional care (Cornelius et al., 2011).

Jones et al. (2011) examined the integration of CBT and MI in the treatment of co-occurring substance use and bipolar disorder. Through a collection of five individual case studies, Jones et al. (2011) concluded that integrated motivational interviewing and cognitive-behavioral therapy for comorbid substance use and bipolar disorder are "feasible and acceptable." Researchers report they determined changes in substance use, often despite participants not reporting it initially as a primary therapy target. They also claim these reductions were typically still present at six-month follow-up.

A study conducted by Baker et al. (2006) that considered a 10-session intervention consisting of CBT and MI in reducing substance use and improving symptomology and general functioning of people with psychotic disorders and comorbid depression found short-term improvement in depression and a similar trend in the reduction of cannabis use. "There was no differential benefit of the intervention on substance use at 12 months, except for a potentially clinically important effect on amphetamine use" (Baker et al., 2006).

Little information was found linking Dialectical Behavior Therapy (DBT) to co-occurring disorders. Some research exists linking DBT to borderline personality disorder (BPD), which Bassir Nia (2018) claims is the second most common personality disorder in patients with substance use disorders, after antisocial personality disorder. While there is no other evidence validating this claim, Bassir Nia (2018) found a 24–56% comorbidity rate for borderline personality disorder co-occurring with substance use disorders.

A study by Stepp et al. (2008) reported a "significant reduction" in self-harm when borderline personality disorder symptoms were measured pre- and post-treatment by the PAI-BOR (Personal Assessment Inventory-Borderline Scale). A reduction in self-harm, which included a measure of impulsivity, is often linked to substance use.

A systemic review of interventions for co-occurring substance use disorders and borderline personality disorders conducted by Pennay et al. (2011) reported DBT with replacement medications effectively reduced substance use and retained participants in treatment over the 12-month period. The participants demonstrated significant reduction in opiate use over the first 30 days of care (Pennay et al., 2011). The researchers also reported that DBT recipients demonstrated no difference in opioid use at 16 months when compared to the participants in the study who received CVT-12S (Comprehensive Validation Therapy with 12-step).

Another practice approach appearing in this review was the mindfulness and self-awareness aspect of DBT as key in this therapy. Mindfulness Oriented Recovery Enhancement (MORE) involves mindfulness training to target automatic habit behavior and foster nonreactivity (Garland et al., 2016). MORE includes reappraisal training to regulate negative emotions and instill a sense of meaningfulness.

Garland et al. (2016) considered substance dependence, traumatic stress, and psychiatric disorders. Client training involved mindful breathing and body scan techniques with an emphasis on developing metacognitive awareness. The process of interrupting the automatic emotional reaction and facilitating cognitive reappraisal may have led to the observed reduction in post-traumatic stress (Garland et al., 2016). Mindfulness promotes positive reappraisals of life adversity to enhance post-traumatic growth and well-being. MORE is associated with significant improvements in positive and negative affect and in symptoms of depression and anxiety (Garland et al., 2016).

A study by Bowen et al. (2014) examined mindfulness-based relapse prevention therapy. This study compared treatment as usual (TAU), consisting of 12-step programming and psychoeducation with relapse prevention therapy (RP) and mindfulness-based relapse prevention therapy (MBRP). Mindfulness practices in this study, much like the MORE technique (Garland et al., 2016), identify individual risk factors and common antecedents of relapse. This practice also increased awareness of and exposure to emotional and cognitive experience and increased awareness of behavioral flexibility (Bowen et al., 2014). Researchers reported 31% fewer days of heavy drinking compared to those who received TAU at 6 months and 31% fewer drug use days and a significantly higher probability of not engaging in heavy drinking at 12 months (Bowen et al., 2014).

Level and Intensity of Care

Limited data was found regarding outcomes of the various treatment modalities (i.e., inpatient, residential, intensive outpatient, etc.). The literature does suggest a consensus that the quality of the treatment plan, the therapy method used, and the skill of the clinician contribute more to the recovery than does the modality (Johnson, 2004).

McCarty et al. (2014) used a combination of randomized trials and naturalistic analysis to compare intensive outpatient care (IOP) to inpatient care, claiming that both service modalities demonstrated comparable outcomes. Drake, O'Neal, and Wallach (2017) suggest that their research indicated the three most effective elements of integrated treatment included group counseling, contingency management, and long-term residential treatment.

In a report on clinician practices, Wendt and Gone (2017) determined an underappreciated dimension of the research-practice gap for substance use disorder treatment is a focus of clinical research on individual therapy. This study determined the prominent modality for co-occurring disordered clients is group therapy, specifically open groups (Wendt & Gone, 2017).

Clearly, more research must be done to determine which treatment modality provides the most effective venue for clients with co-occurring disorders. While much of the outcome research cited here focused on treatment models, primarily Cognitive Behavioral Therapy and Motivational Interviewing, questions remain about where best to locate services and when inpatient and/or residential care may be required versus intensive outpatient or outpatient care (see Quadrants of Care above). The other issue that seems overlooked in the current literature is the efficacy of community 12-step support groups as part of a continuum of care. In the substance use field, attendance by clients at these programs has been a hallmark of treatment. Given the new realities of co-occurring disorders, it would be helpful to learn if these groups are effective with substance abuse clients experiencing mental health challenges as well.

BEST-PRACTICE TREATMENT RECOMMENDATIONS

From a treatment perspective, clients with co-occurring disorders exhibit and experience more severe and chronic medical, social, and emotional problems (SAMHSA, 2005) and are more difficult to engage in assessment and treatment

(Johnson, 2004; Denning, 2000). Profiles of clients with co-occurring disorders consistently demonstrate they require more services than clients with a single issue. Because these clients have at least two disorders, they are vulnerable to both substance use relapse and a worsening of the mental health condition. Further, relapse with substances often leads to psychiatric decompensation, and worsening of psychiatric symptoms often leads to relapse with substances. Hence, relapse prevention treatment must be specially designed for clients with co-occurring disorders (see below).

Clients with a co-occurring disorder often have more crises and progress more gradually in treatment. These clients have higher rates of homelessness and legal and medical problems, often needing more frequent and longer-lasting hospitalizations and have more frequent emergency room visits (SAMHSA, 2005). For example, clients with schizophrenia are twice as likely to experience episodes of violence and suicide if they simultaneously abuse street drugs (Anthony, Warner, & Kessler, 1997).

The treatment and social needs of clients with co-occurring disorders differ depending on the type and severity of the disorders. They are less able to navigate between, engage in, and remain engaged in treatment services (Johnson, 2004). Therefore, treatment must be suited to the client's personal needs and characteristics, often across the various treatment systems. Moreover, abstinence from substance use may not be appropriate for these clients, suggesting that a harm reduction approach instead of a disease model approach may be more appropriate (SAMHSA, 2005).

The prevailing attitudes and beliefs about how to best treat clients with co-occurring disorders are changing. As the substance abuse and mental health fields become increasingly aware that clients with co-occurring disorders require adaptation and flexibility in traditional ideas and methods, various attempts have been made to account for the special needs of this population (Baker, 1991; Minkoff & Drake, 1991; Ries, 1993). As a professional practitioner interested in treating substance abusing clients, clients with mental illness, or both, understanding how to provide treatment to this complex and significantly at-risk population is important.

According to Baker (1991), these attempts reflect philosophical differences between substance and mental health fields about the nature of co-occurring disorders, as well as differing opinions regarding the best way to treat them. While the evidence demonstrated earlier suggests these attitudes are changing, more progress is needed. The limitations on integrated treatment also reflect the limitations of available resources and differences in treatment responses for different types and severities of problems.

An integrated model of treatment combines elements of both substance abuse and mental health treatments into a unified and comprehensive treatment program designed specifically for clients with co-occurring disorders (SAMHSA, 2005).

In this model, professionals are cross-trained in substance use and mental health assessment and treatments and often utilize case management as a way of monitoring and supporting clients through various substance abuse and mental health crises as they occur. One provider or program provides the primary treatment for both the substance abuse and mental health problems simultaneously as part of a comprehensive treatment approach. If outside services are required, such as psychiatric evaluation and medication, vocational counseling, credit counseling, or legal services, the primary provider serves in the role of case manager, seeing to it that the client receives the services they require as part of the overall comprehensive treatment approach (Evans & Sullivan, 2001).

From the professional literature and clinical experience, below is a list of best-practice issues to consider when treating persons with co-occurring substance abuse problems and mental health disorders. Keep in mind these issues must be considered in the context of other groups and communities of which the client is a member or associates with in their life (i.e., racial, ethnic, age, sexual orientation, etc.). In the context of an integrated treatment approach discussed above, please consider the following:

1. **Focus on building trusting, respectful, and supportive relationships.** From Chapter 1 in this text, successful treatment is built on this foundation. Before treatment models or interventions can work, clients must have an investment in the therapeutic relationship as something they value.
2. **Always keep the First Practice Principle in front of your mind.** In Chapter 1, we discussed at length the value of the First Practice Principle in helping clients make long-term connections to helpful and supportive systems. The research discussed above bears this out. As a reminder, the First Practice Principle states: Healthy outcomes (and lives) are directly related to people's connections to helpful, supportive systems across a lifetime.
3. **Employ Culturally Respectful and Appropriate methods.** See Chapter 1 for the importance and value of being culturally appropriate in client engagement.
4. **Accurate and comprehensive assessment and diagnoses are critical** (SAMHSA, 2005; Johnson, 2004). Professionals must acquire training in substance use, mental health, and different modalities (i.e., group and family therapy) where best-practice treatment occurs.
5. **Dual recovery approach** (SAMHSA, 2005; Evans & Sullivan, 2001). This approach can best be described as a recovery-oriented approach for both the substance use and mental health disorder. According to Evans and Sullivan (2001),

> The priority for early stages of recovery from chemical dependency is simply maintaining abstinence, and

typically, the interventions rely on frequent AA meetings ... Later chemical dependency work relies on step work to achieve positive aspects of health through addressing issues such as guilt, fear, and resentment. Similarly, the priority in the early stages of recovery from psychiatric disorders is simply maintaining stability, and typically, interventions rely on case management, a structured lifestyle, and acceptance of the need to manage the disorder. Later mental health work relies on skills training and psychotherapy to achieve positive functioning through addressing issues such as grief at having an illness, establishing intimacy, and operating as a prosocial member of society. (p. 29)

6. **Motivational enhancement through Motivational Interviewing.** As we discussed in Chapter 1 and demonstrated through the literature in this chapter, focusing clients on their stage of change for each diagnosed problem (substance use and mental health) and using motivational interviewing (Miller & Rollnick, 2002) to help clients enhance their motivation to change are part of an important well-documented positive skill set in this field (SAMHSA, 2005).

7. **Use an "Illness" Metaphor/Model as a foundation for treatment.** For many persons with co-occurring disorders, thinking about their "illness" provides clients with a nonjudgmental rationale for the need to abstain from substances and is a way for practitioners to help clients reframe their sense of self from troubled to "ill." Simultaneously, this approach reinforces education about the nature of their mental health disorder. It also provides a long-term and consistent mechanism to help guard against relapse, and it allows clients an opportunity to explore the existential and spiritual issues that persons with co-occurring disorder often face in the context of illness, instead of more stigmatizing definitions of self they often face in their daily life.

8. **Employ CBT in individual, group, and family treatment.** Clients with co-occurring disorders are treated in individual, group, and family therapy. According to Evans and Sullivan (2001) and the latest evidence described above, a cognitive-behavioral approach combined with Motivational Interviewing (Miller & Rollnick, 2002) is currently most effective in each of the three modalities. CBT focuses on thinking and action and are especially good at relapse prevention and teaching new coping mechanisms for life stressors (SAMHSA, 2005).

9. **Attend to the basics first.** Attend to your client's most immediate crisis first before moving into treatment. That is, look for potential emotional,

psychological, or physical issues early in your contact to ensure your client has their needs met by the appropriate professional. After these issues have been stabilized and addressed, formal treatment planning to address the co-occurring disorders can begin. Think of this as a "practice hierarchy of needs" that encompasses, food, clothing, shelter, health, and safety. Without these issues stabilized, it is difficult to get clients to work on their other issues in good faith.

10. **Focus on relapse prevention.** Relapse is a common occurrence in substance abuse treatment. So common that many suggest it should become a conscious part of treatment dialogue very early in the process (Gorski, 1990; 1992; 1993; Gorski & Miller, 1986), while others believe that discussing relapse can trigger a relapse (Evans & Sullivan, 2001).

   Whatever the strategy one takes toward relapse, research consistently finds upward of 70% relapse (substances) within the first year after primary treatment (Johnson, 2004; Fisher & Harrison, 2000). As discussed earlier, a substance relapse can have devastating effects on a person with co-occurring disorders, including medication/substances interaction leading to overdoses, exacerbation of mental health symptoms, and treatment dropout. Moreover, practitioners can use the same language and tactics to discuss potential mental health relapses as well (i.e., stop taking meds, ignoring newly learned coping skills to manage symptoms, etc.). Here is a simple guide to relapse prevention (Johnson, 2004):

   - **Determine high-risk situations.** What circumstances place clients at high risk for relapse? This involves identifying triggers in the environment and in the client's way of thinking that begin the process of their triggers and cravings overwhelming them.
   - **Develop strategies to cope with high-risk situations.** Once identified, clients must develop coping strategies. Group treatment is helpful in this step, as clients can share experiences and strategies in a supportive and helpful manner. However, one can be just as successful during individual therapy, too. Focus on teaching clients alternative ways to handle high-risk situations by giving homework that forces clients to practice these responses.
   - **Social support is critical.** Help clients engage and remain in positive social support networks such as AA or NA, church, groups of supportive friends, and/or family. Group treatment is helpful in this area, as it exposes clients to new, supportive networks. Family treatment can also be helpful in this regard.
   - **Holistic approach to relapse prevention.** Any approach to relapse prevention must take a multi-system, holistic approach to be successful over the long term. This includes issues related to individual activities

(recreation, relationships, health), family, and their local environment. Think about and ask what clients like to do for fun. Treatment cannot be serious all the time. Outside hobbies, recreation, and enjoyment can help build momentum for long-term change.
- **Make a discussion about the relapse part of treatment.** The goal of relapse prevention is to: (1) keep the amount and duration of the relapse contained; (2) lengthen the time between relapses; (3) help clients place relapses into a positive context; and (4) retain clients in treatment after relapses occur.

To accomplish these goals, it is appropriate to begin discussing the probability of relapse early in treatment, along with efforts to reframe a relapse as a normal and regular part of the recovery process (i.e., two steps forward, one step back). It is vital you do not give clients the impression a relapse signals failure, the loss of all that has been gained, or a disappointment to yourself or anyone else. If clients come to accept relapses as a normal part of the process, the four goals stated earlier can be met with minimal damage to the client's sense of self or level of self-efficacy.

11. **Quadrants of Care.** Review the Quadrants of Care discussion earlier in this chapter, based on the severity of each client disorder. This conceptualization of treatment needs based on severity can prove helpful. Given that most agencies and organizations do not meet the definition of Integrated Care, this level system offers practitioners a guide for meeting client needs, depending on their symptom presentation and the practitioner's location in either the substance abuse or mental health system.

To close, we return to Chapter 1. In that chapter, we presented a one-paragraph statement about our Core Beliefs of practice, both with co-occurring disorders specifically and other clients. Our Core Beliefs, repeated below, encapsulate all we have learned about the current best practices with persons with co-occurring disorders.

CORE BELIEFS

Clients do not change because of models, methods, or interventions alone. They change because they are helped into a trusting and respectful therapeutic relationship based on enhancing their dignity as human beings, have hope they can change for the better, and the motivation to endure the process of change. All of this is accomplished in the context of helpful and supportive systems of support to build personal resilience.

REFERENCES

American Psychological Association. (2018). *Diagnostic and statistical manual* (5th ed.). Author.

Anthony, J. C., Warner, L. A., & Kessler, R. C. (1997). Comparative epidemiology of dependence on tobacco, alcohol, controlled substances, and inhalants: Basic findings from the national comorbidity survey. In G. A. Marlatt & G. R. VandenBos (Eds.), *Addictive behaviors: Readings on etiology, prevention, and treatment* (pp. 3–39). American Psychological Association.

Back, S. E., Brady, K. T., Sonne, S. C., & Verduin, M. L. (2006). Symptom improvement in co-occurring PTSD and alcohol dependence. *The Journal of Nervous and Mental Disease, 194*(9): 690–696.

Baker, A., Bucci, S., Lewin, T. J., Kay-Lambkin, F., Constable, P. M., & Carr, V. J. (2006). Cognitive-behavioural therapy for substance use disorders in people with psychotic disorders: Randomized controlled trial. *The British Journal of Psychiatry, 188*(5): 439–448.

Baker, A. L., Hales, S. A., Thornton, L. K., Hides, L., & Lubman, D. I. (2012). A systematic review of psychological interventions for excessive alcohol consumption among people with psychotic disorders. *Acta Psychiatrica Scandinavica, 126*(4): 243–255.

Baker, F. (1991). *Coordination of alcohol, drug abuse, and mental health services* (TIP #4). Office of Treatment Improvement, Alcohol, Drug Abuse, and Mental Health Administration.

Bassir Nia, A. (2018). Opioid addiction and borderline personality disorder. *The American Journal on Addictions, 27*(1): 54–55.

Bowen, S., Witkiewitz, K., Clifasefi, S. L., Grow, J., Chawla, N., Hsu, S. H., & Larimer, M. E. (2014). Relative efficacy of mindfulness-based relapse prevention, standard relapse prevention, and treatment as usual for substance use disorders: A randomized clinical trial. *JAMA Psychiatry, 71*(5): 547–556.

Brook, R. C., & Whitehead, P. C. (1980). *Drug-free therapeutic community: An evaluation.* Human Sciences Press.

Brown, R. A., Evans, M., Miller, I. W., Burgess, E. S., & Mueller, T. I. (1997). Cognitive-behavioral treatment for depression in alcoholism. *Journal of Consulting and Clinical Psychology 7*(65): 715–726.

Chen, S., Barnett, P. G., Sempel, J. M., & Timko, C. (2006). Outcomes and costs of matching the intensity of dual-diagnosis treatment to patients' symptom severity. *Journal of Substance Abuse Treatment, 31*: 95–105.

Compton, W. M., Cottler, L. B., Jacobs, J. L., Ben-Abdallah, A., & Spitznagel, E. L. (2003). The role of psychiatric disorders in predicting drug dependence treatment outcomes. *American Journal of Psychiatry, 160*: 890–895.

Compton, W. M. III, Cottler, L. B., Ben Abdallah, A., Phelps, D. L., Spitznagel, E. L., & Horton, J. C. (2000). Substance dependence and other psychiatric disorders among drug dependent subjects: Race and gender correlates. *American Journal of Addictions 9*(2): 113–125.

Cornelius, J. R., Douaihy, A., Bukstein, O. G., Daley, D. C., Wood, S. D., Kelly, T. M., & Salloum, I. M. (2011). Evaluation of cognitive behavioral therapy/motivational enhancement therapy (CBT/MET) in a treatment trial of comorbid MDD/AUD adolescents. *Addictive Behaviors, 36*(8): 843–848.

Crome, I. B. (1999). Substance misuse and psychiatric comorbidity: Towards improved service provision. *Drugs: Education, Prevention & Policy 6*(2): 151–174.

Curran, G. M., Kirchner, J. E., Worley, M., Rookey, C., & Booth, B. M. (2002). Depressive symptomatology and early attrition from intensive outpatient substance use treatment. *Journal of Behavioral Health Services & Research 29*: 138–143.

De Leon, G. (1989). Psychopathology and substance abuse: What is being learned from research in therapeutic communities. *Journal of Psychoactive Drugs 21*(2): 177–188.

De Leon, G. (1984). *The therapeutic community: Study of effectiveness.* National Institute on Drug Abuse.

De Leon, G., & Jainchill, N. (1982). Male and female drug abusers: Social and psychological status after treatment in a therapeutic community. *American Journal of Drug and Alcohol Abuse 8*: 464–497.

Denning, P. (2000). *Practicing harm reduction psychotherapy: An alternative approach to addictions.* Guilford Press.

Donald, M., Dower, J., & Kavanagh, D. (2005). Integrated versus non-integrated management and care for clients with co-occurring systematic review of randomized controlled trials. *Social Sciences & Medicine, 60*: 1371–1383.

Drake, R. E., Mercer-McFadden, C., Mueser, K. T., McHugo, G. J., & Bond, G. R. (1998). Review of integrated mental health and substance abuse treatment for patients with dual disorders. *Schizophrenia Bulletin 24*(4): 589–608.

Drake, R. E., Mueser, K. T., Brunette, M. F., & McHugo, G. J. (2004). A review of treatments for people with severe mental illnesses and co-occurring substance use disorders. *Psychiatric Rehabilitation Journal, 27*: 360–374.

Drake, R. E., O'Neal, E. L., & Wallach, M. A. (2008). A systematic review of psychosocial research on psychosocial interventions for people with co-occurring severe mental and substance use disorders. *Journal of Substance Abuse Treatment, 34*(1): 123–138.

Drake, R. E., Wallach, M. A., & McGovern, M. P. (2005). Future directions in preventing relapse to substance abuse among clients with severe mental illnesses. *Psychiatric Services, 56*: 1297–1302.

Evans, K., & Sullivan, J. M. (2001). *Dual diagnosis: Counseling the mentally ill substance abuser* (2nd ed.). Guilford Press.

Fisher, G. L., & Harrison, T. C. (2000). *Substance abuse: Information for school counselors, social workers, therapists, and counselors* (2nd ed.). Allyn & Bacon.

Flynn, P. M., & Brown, B. S. (2008). Co-occurring disorders in substance abuse treatment: Issues and prospects. *Substance Abuse Treatment* (2008 January) *34*(1): 36–47.

Garland, E. L., Roberts-Lewis, A., Tronnier, C. D., Graves, R., & Kelley, K. (2016). Mindfulness-oriented recovery enhancement versus CBT for co-occurring substance dependence, traumatic stress, and psychiatric disorders: Proximal outcomes from a pragmatic randomized trial. *Behaviour Research and Therapy, 77*: 7–16.

Gorski, T. T. (1990). The Cenaps model of relapse prevention: Basic principles and procedures. *Journal of Psychoactive Drugs, 22*: 125–133.

Gorski, T. T. (1992). Creating a relapse prevention program in your treatment center. *Addiction & Recovery*, July/August: 16–17.

Gorski, T. T. (1993). Relapse prevention: A state of the art overview. *Addiction & Recovery*, March/April: 25–27.

Gorski, T. T., & Miller, M. M. (1986). *Staying sober: Guide to relapse prevention*. Herald House.

Grella, C. E, Joshi, V., & Hser, Y. (2003). Followup of cocaine-dependent men and women with antisocial personality disorder. *Journal of Substance Abuse Treatment 25*: 155–164.

Harris, K. M., & Edlund, M. J. (2005). Use of mental health care and substance abuse treatment among adults with cooccurring disorders. *Psychiatric Services, 56*: 954–959.

Hasin D., Trautman, K., & Endicott, J. (1998). Psychiatric research interview for substance and mental disorders: Phenomenologically based diagnosis in patients who abuse alcohol or drugs. *Psychopharmacology Bulletin 34*: 3–8.

Hides, L. M., Elkins, K. S., Scaffidi, A., Cotton, S. M., Carroll, S., & Lubman, D. I. (2011). Does the addition of integrated cognitive behaviour therapy and motivational interviewing improve the outcomes of standard care for young people with comorbid depression and substance misuse? *Medical Journal of Australia, 195*(3): S31–S37.

Hien, D. A., Cohen, L. R., Miele, G. M., Litt, L. C., & Capstick, C. (2004). Promising treatments for women with comorbid PTSD and substance use disorders. *American Journal of Psychiatry 161*: 1426–1432.

Hien, D. A., Jiang, H., Campbell, A. N. C., Hu, M., Miele, G. M., Cohen, L. R., & Nunes, E. V. (2010). Do treatment improvements in PTSD severity affect substance use outcomes? A secondary analysis from a randomized analysis from a randomized clinical trial in NIDA's clinical trials network. *The American Journal of Psychiatry, 167*(1): 95–101.

Hser, Y. I., Grella, C., Evans, E., & Huang, Y. C. (2006). Utilization and outcomes of mental health services among patients in drug treatment. *Journal of Addictive Diseases 25*: 73–85.

Hser, Y., Grella, C., Hubbard, R. L., Hsieh, S., Fletcher, B. W., Brown, B. S., & Anglin, M. D. (2001). An evaluation of drug treatment for adolescents in 4 US cities. *Archives of General Psychiatry, 58*: 689–695.

Hubbard, R. L., Marsden, M. E., Rachal, J. V., Harwood, H. J., Cavanaugh, E. R., & Ginzburg, H. M. (1989). *Drug abuse treatment: A national study of effectiveness.* University of North Carolina Press.

Hunter, S. B., Watkins, K. E., Hepner, K. A., Paddock, S. M., Ewing Osilla, K. C., & Perry, S. (2012). Treating depression and substance use: A randomized controlled trial. *Journal of Substance Abuse Treatment, 43*(2): 137–151.

Joe, G. W., Brown, B. S., & Simpson, D. (1995). Psychological problems and client engagement in methadone treatment. *Journal of Nervous and Mental Disease, 183*(11): 704–710.

Johnson, J. L. (2004). *Fundamentals of substance abuse practice.* Wadsworth/Brooks/Cole.

Jones, S. H., Barrowclough, C., Allott, R., Day, C., Earnshaw, P., & Wilson, I. (2011). Integrated motivational interviewing and cognitive-behavioural therapy for bipolar disorder with comorbid substance use: Integrated MI and CBT for bipolar disorder. *Clinical Psychology & Psychotherapy, 18*(5): 426–437.

Karageorge, K. (2001). Treatment Benefits the Mental Health of Adolescents, Young Adults, and Adults. NEDS Fact Sheet 78. National Evaluation Data Services.

Killeen, T. K., Back, S. E., & Brady, K. T. (2015). Implementation of integrated therapies for comorbid post-traumatic stress disorder and substance use disorders in community substance abuse treatment programs. *Drug and Alcohol Review, 34*(3): 234–241.

McCarty, D., Braude, L., Lyman, D. R., Dougherty, R. H., Daniels, A. S., Ghose, S. S., & Delphin-Rittmon, M. E. (2014). Substance abuse intensive outpatient programs: Assessing the evidence. *Psychiatric Services, 65*(6): 718.

McGovern, M. P., Lambert-Harris, C., Acquilano, S., Xie, H., Alterman, A. I., & Weiss, R. D. (2009). A cognitive behavioral therapy for co-occurring substance use and posttraumatic stress disorders. *Addictive Behaviors, 34*(10): 892–897.

McGovern, M. P., Lambert-Harris, C., Alterman, A. I., Xie, H., & Meier, A. (2011). A randomized controlled trial comparing integrated cognitive behavioral therapy versus individual addiction counseling for co-occurring substance use and post-traumatic stress disorders. *Journal of Dual Diagnosis, 7*(4): 207–227.

Menezes, P. R., Johnson, S., Thornicraft, G., Marshall, L., Prosser, D., Bennington, P., & Kuipers, E. (1996). Drug and alcohol problems among individuals with severe mental illness in South London. *British Journal of Psychiatry, 168*(5): 612–619.

Miller, W. R., & Rollnick, S. (2002). *Motivational interviewing: Preparing people to change addictive behavior* (2nd ed.). Guilford Press.

Minkoff, K., & Drake, R. E., Eds. (1991). *Dual diagnosis of major mental illness and substance disorder.* Jossey-Bass.

Mueser, K. T., Torrey, W. C., & Lynde, D. (2003). Implementing evidence-based practices for people with severe mental illness (Special issue: Empirically supported treatments). *Behavior Modification, 27*: 387–411.

Nace, E. P, & Davis, C. W. (1993). Treatment outcome in substance abusing patients with a personality disorder. *American Journal of Addiction 2*: 26–33.

Office of the Surgeon General. (1999). *Mental Health: A Report of the Surgeon General.* US Public Health Service.

Osher, F. C. (1996). A vision for the future: Toward a service system responsive to those with co-occurring addictive and mental disorders. *American Journal of Orthopsychiatry, 66*: 71–76.

Pennay, A., Cameron, J., Reichert, T., Strickland, H., Lee, N. K., Hall, K., & Lubman, D. I. (2011). A systematic review of interventions for co-occurring substance use disorder and borderline personality disorder. *Journal of Substance Abuse Treatment, 41*(4), 363–373.

Pepper, B., Kirshner, M. C., & Ryglewicz, H. (1981). The young adult chronic patient: Overview of a population. *Hospital and Community Psychiatry 32*(7):463–469.

Ries, R. K. The dually diagnosed patient with psychotic symptoms. *Journal of Addictive Diseases, 12*(3): 103–122.

Riper, H., Andersson, G., Hunter, S. B., De Wit, J., Berking, M., & Cuijpers, P. (2014). Treatment of comorbid alcohol use disorders and depression with cognitive-behavioural therapy and motivational interviewing: A meta-analysis. *Addiction, 109*(3): 394–421.

Ross, S., Dermatis, H., Levounis, P., & Galanter, M. (2003). A comparison between dually diagnosed inpatients with and without Axis II comorbidity and the relationship to treatment outcomes. *American Journal of Drug and Alcohol Abuse, 29*: 263–279.

Rounsaville, B. J., Weissman, M. M., Kleber, H., & Wilber, C. (1982). Heterogeneity of psychiatric diagnosis in treated opiate addicts. *Archives of General Psychiatry, 39*(2): 161–168.

SAMHSA (n.d.) Definition retrieved from: https://store.samhsa.gov/system/files/sma13-3992.pdf

SAMHSA (2005). *Substance abuse treatment for persons with co-occurring disorders: A treatment improvement protocol, 42.* US Department of Health and Human Services.

Sciacca, K. (1991). Integrated treatment approach for severely mentally ill individuals with substance disorders. *New Directions for Mental Health Services, 50*: 69–84.

Simpson, D. D., Joe, G. W., & Broome, K. M. (2002). A national 5-year follow-up of treatment outcomes for cocaine dependence. *Archives of General Psychiatry, 59*: 538–544.

Stepp, S., Epler, A., Jahng, S., & Trull, T. (2008). The effect of dialectical behavior therapy skills use on borderline personality disorder features. *Journal of Personality Disorders, 22*(6): 549–563.

Quello, S. B., Brady, K. T., & Sonne, S. C. (2005). Mood disorders and substance use disorders: A complex comorbidity. *Science and Practice Perspectives,* (3): 13–24.

Watkins, K. E., Burnam, A., Kung, F. Y., & Paddock, S. (2001). A national survey of care for persons with co-occurring mental and substance use disorders. *Psychiatric Services, 52*(8): 1062–1068.

Watkins, K. E., Hunter, S. B., Burnam, M. A., Pincus, H. A., & Nicholson, G. (2005). Review of treatment recommendations for persons with a co-occurring affective or anxiety and substance use disorder. *Psychiatric Services, 56*(8): 913–926.

Weathers, F. W., Ruscio, A. M., & Keane, T. M. (1999). Psychometric properties of nine scoring rules for the clinician-administered posttraumatic stress disorder scale. *Psychological Assessment, 11*(2): 124–133.

Wendt, D. C., & Gone, J. P. (2017). Group therapy for substance use disorders: A survey of clinician practices. *Journal of Groups in Addiction & Recovery, 12*(4): 243–259.

Woody, G. E., & Blaine, J. (1979). Depression in narcotic addicts: Quite possibly more than a chance association. In R. L. Dupont, A. Goldstein, J. O'Donnell, & B. Brown B. (Eds.), *Handbook on Drug Abuse.* US Government Printing Office, 277-285.

Woody, G. E., McLellan, A. T., O'Brien, C. P., & Luborsky, L. (1991). Addressing psychiatric comorbidity. In R. W. Picken, C. G. Leukefeld, & C. R. Schuster (Eds.), *Improving Drug Abuse Treatment.* NIDA Research Monograph 106. National Institute on Drug Abuse, pp. 152–166.

ABOUT THE EDITORS

Jerry L. Johnson, Ph.D., MSW is an associate professor in the School of Social Work at Grand Valley State University in Grand Rapids, Michigan. He received his MSW from Grand Valley State University and his Ph.D. in sociology from Western Michigan University. Johnson has been in the human services field since 1983, serving as a family therapist, clinical supervisor, administrator, consultant, teacher, trainer, and author. He was the recipient of two Fulbright Scholarship awards to Albania in 1998-99 and 2000-01. In addition to teaching and writing, Johnson serves in various consulting capacities in countries such as Albania, Armenia, and China.

He is the author of two previous books, Crossing Borders—Confronting History: Intercultural Adjustment in a Post-Cold War World (2000, Rowan and Littlefield) and Fundamentals of Substance Abuse Practice (2004, Wadsworth Brooks/Cole).

George Grant, Jr., Ph.D., LMSW is the dean of the College of Community and Public Service and a professor in the School of Social Work at Grand Valley State University in Grand Rapids, Michigan. He received his BSW from Marygrove College, MSW from Grand Valley State University, and Ph.D. in sociology from Western Michigan University. Grant, Jr. is a professor, administrator, evaluator, practitioner, consultant, and committed to community engagement primary in the fields of child welfare.

Dr. Johnson and Dr. Grant are the editors of a previous eight-volume casebook series, including: Substance Abuse (2005), Mental Health (2005), Foster Care (2005), Adoption (2005), Domestic Violence (2005), Community Practice (2005), Medical Social Work (2005), and Sexual Abuse (2007).

ABOUT THE AUTHORS

Jerry L. Johnson, PhD provided direct clinical services to clients with a range of co-occurring disorders for more than 15 years. He continues to be a popular clinical consultant and trainer, specifically pertaining to substance use disorders and trauma. Along with Dr. George Grant, Jr., he is a co-editor of the present casebook series.

Salvador Lopez-Arias, PhD is an Associate Professor in the School of Social Work at Grand Valley State University. He received a PhD in Counseling Psychology from Western Michigan University and his MSW from Grand Valley State University. Lopez-Arias has been a practitioner for 28 years with a broad focus. His clinical work has focused on culturally competent practice in co-occurring disorders, trauma, family therapy, and holistic health, with an emphasis in substance use disorders. He is also involved in the areas of community engagement, evaluation, and research.

Carolyn Sutherby received her MSW from Grand Valley State University and her PhD in Social Work from Michigan State University. She has been working in the human services field since 1998. Sutherby has worked as a clinical therapist providing treatment to children and adolescents, adults, and couples. She specializes in treating women with behavioral health issues and trauma histories who are involved in the criminal justice and child welfare systems. Sutherby trains clinicians and direct service providers on working with mothers who have survived trauma. She has also consulted with organizations on creating gender-responsive, trauma-informed, and clinically sound programming.

Glen A. Brookhouse, LLMSW is a graduate of Grand Valley State University. Beginning in 2015, he focused his social work studies in the area of homelessness and substance use disorders. Since that time, he has been employed as a counselor and advocate for homeless individuals. He completed his graduate studies as a Recovery Management Substance Abuse Therapist at Family Outreach Center in Grand Rapids, Michigan. His position gives him the opportunity to provide substance use disorder services to individuals experiencing poverty and homelessness.

CPSIA information can be obtained
at www.ICGtesting.com
Printed in the USA
BVHW051925280821
615383BV00006B/123